Fresh Start Cworkbook

A personalized guide to making baby food at home.

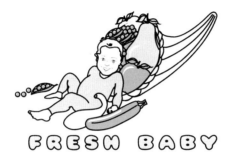

This book belongs to

_____

Caution:

Published by Fresh Baby LLC
357 East 57th Street, New York, NY 10022
www.myfreshbaby.com

Library of Congress Cataloging-in-Publication Data is available.

To purchase additional copies of this book or to learn more about Fresh Baby's other products, visit our
web site at www.myfreshbaby.com or call 866-403-7374

Authors: Joan Ahlers and Cheryl Tallman

Cover and Interior Book Design: Emilya Naymark—www.emmawest.com
Editors: Laurel Davis and Alison Tartt
Print in Korea by asianprinting.com

To our parents, Al and Charlotte Moellenbeck, for all the love, support, and caring you give us. Without it we would not be the people we are today. A special thank you to Mom for teaching us how to cook and providing expert advice on the recipes in this book. Thanks for everything. We love you!

To our wonderful and loving husbands, Roger Tallman and Gary Ahlers, for allowing us the time and giving us the support and encouragement to make Fresh Baby a reality.

The Fresh Start Kit is dedicated to our own Fresh Babies—Spencer Tallman, Madison, Jordan, Gregory, and Sienna Ahlers. We are trying to give you the best start in life and hope that you will grow up to make a difference in the beautiful world that we live in.

Joan Ahlers

Cheryl Tallman

Contents

A Father's Tale

pparently my wife was a total research nut. Our countertops and tables were a flurry of measuring cups, mixtures, and notes. I quickly discovered the advantage in being an insider to this process. Thanks to Cheryl's investigative skill and the talent and experience of her accomplice and sister, Joanie, babies and their dads have a great foundation for the very first journey into solid food. Cheryl and Joanie started with their personal experiences of making baby food for five babies and then studied up on what's really good for babies and on proper nutrition. And best of all, they invited me to help in the preparation one night.

Our home had turned into a test kitchen.

I really didn't know what to expect. Cheryl picked out sweet potatoes and apples for a few starter meals for our baby, Spencer. Sounded good to me. As we washed and peeled, she filled me in on all the things you need to know about food, and how it gets from the farms to the market. She had some frightening things to say, and other things that made a lot of sense, such as washing your food really well to get the pesticides and dirt off. This was standard practice in my family because both of my parents grew up on farms. Then everything in our kitchen began to smell wonderful. It felt like we were in the country. The fragrance of apples permeated our apartment. What we were doing felt great. It just felt right. Right for our kid and, you know, the educated parental thing to do. I was diggin' it! We went through all the steps in the Fresh Baby process in no time. It took us less than an hour to finish making two weeks of food for our baby. I felt very proud about doing something good for Spencer. Fresh Baby was actually quite easy and I was about to find out how easily it worked on kids. The next morning was a morning that Cheryl had asked me to get up with Spencer so she could get a little extra sleep.

Breakfast is a breeze.

Spencer is very vocal in the morning. He wants you to know that it's time for everybody to get up. As soon as the sun comes in the window, we hear the familiar baby sounds, the universal signal calling all parents that means, "Get up. It's my time now." After cooking with Cheryl, answering that wake-up call has become easier. Now when I reach the kitchen at 7:00 a.m., it's a conscious experience. And I find I have a new relationship with the freezer. I know it's my friend because I'll find good-tasting and nutritious choices for my kid's breakfast. I also know that when breakfast is all over, he has a great start on the day. He's happy with what he tastes, and he's having a good time eating.

My special "best bet" Saturday breakfast (for 7-month-olds) includes:

- 2 frozen Fresh Baby fruit cubes (peaches and pears)
- 2 scoops of oatmeal baby cereal with a little soy formula mixed in
- And to finish everything off—about 5 ounces of formula

Mealtimes these days for us are a chance to enjoy the fun of Spencer experiencing these new tastes in his life. Knowing that I'm helping him develop good eating habits that will stay with him forever is very rewarding.

Wow—picking out and making food is much more satisfying than going to the store and just buying jars of baby food. Buying fresh and fresh-frozen is a joy because you know the food is chock full of flavor and vitamins. It's more fulfilling for us, too, because my wife and I have a say about what goes into Spencer's mouth. Besides, it's a real family experience in the supermarket. I see it in his face as all the new sights and sounds stimulate him. All the cool colors. When you think about it, shopping is a basic life experience—and something kids love to share with Dad or Mom. We take Spencer with us and explain the produce and milk departments. He seemed to get the connection early on between bright colors and tasty food. In years to come, these experiences will make a big difference in his eating habits. I think it also helps place food in a healthier perspective.

This little baby goes to the market.

In closing, I hope all parents will try to be a bigger part of what our wonderful kids need. What we do for children in their formative years lasts forever. We are passing on a lifestyle built on the basics of love, support, nurturing, and education. As parents we are teachers. Little things that we commit to ultimately make a big difference in how they view their lives. I am proud to say that Fresh Baby has made it easier for me to know I'm doing my part as a dad. After all, as most of us in charge of budding appetites know well, you are what you eat.

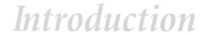

Introduction

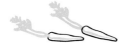

Hi and welcome to Fresh Baby!

As a new parent, you want to provide your baby with the best possible start in life. Studies show that babies who are fed nutritious, healthy diets grow into stronger kids and better-adjusted eaters than those who are fed poor diets. Fresh Baby's Fresh Start Kit is a complete system to help you prepare your baby's food at home and help your baby start smart with good eating habits from the very first bite of solid food.

Fresh Baby's system is unique and specially designed for parents who recognize the benefits of preparing fresh, all-natural baby food but do not have a lot time in their busy schedules. Designed by a working mother, the Fresh Baby system teaches you to make your baby's food quickly and in quantity. The food is frozen in specially designed freezer trays, with each compartment containing a single one-ounce serving. Once it is frozen into food cubes and stored in the freezer, it is always ready to use, easy to transport for your baby's days away from home, and fresh for up to 2 months.

The Fresh Baby Cworkbook is more than just a cookbook. An easy-to-read combination cookbook and workbook, the Cworkbook's first section outlines the essentials of feeding your baby and teaches you how to make nutritious baby food quickly and easily. A second section features Fresh Baby's specially designed recipes. Because cooking—especially for your kids—can be a creative and entertaining process, and because each child is unique, the Cworkbook provides space for recording notes about your baby's feeding patterns and experiences. The first section of the Cworkbook covers these topics:

- Healthy eating habits
- Benefits of home-prepared baby food
- Introducing solid foods
- Dietary essentials for babies
- Making and serving Fresh Baby food
- Kitchen tools
- Safety basics
- Food choices
- Fresh Baby to go
- Managing your time

Organized by baby's age for easy reference, each recipe contains all the information you need to know in order to shop, cook, and serve your baby's food. The recipes contain detailed how-to steps for preparing wholesome food at home as well as other helpful tips and guidelines:

- Ripeness and storage—to help you select and properly store fresh produce
- Nutritional information—provides basic vitamin and mineral content
- Total preparation time—from start to finish you will know how long the recipe takes
- Variations—includes creative ideas for adding herbs, spices, and natural flavors
- Serving—offers examples on tasty and nutritious combinations

Throughout the Cworkbook, we provide space for recording your baby's eating habits and reactions. Jotting down notes and customizing your Cworkbook for your baby's needs makes feedings go easier for you and your baby and helps eliminate the possibility of making the same mistake twice! Use your baby's personalized pages daily, and you'll be creating a keepsake for memories that can be enjoyed time and time again. There are places for fun stories, food likes and dislikes, favorite recipes, and those priceless first-time feeding snapshots.

The Fresh Baby way of preparing baby food is a simple, nutritious, and economical plan that makes it easy for you to make sure your child gets the best start possible. Many people don't realize that making baby food at home has many benefits.

For babies:
- A nutritious and great-tasting introduction to solid food
- Freshness and variety in food choices with elimination of all additives
- The love, attention, and care that is put into making food and feeding times

For parents:
- The satisfaction of knowing that you are doing what is best for your baby
- Control over what your baby eats and how the food is prepared
- Ease, convenience, and cost savings

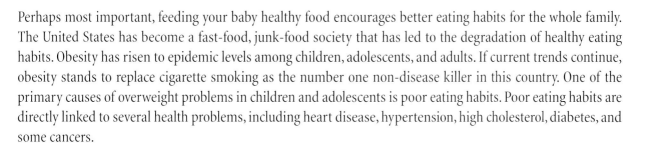

Perhaps most important, feeding your baby healthy food encourages better eating habits for the whole family. The United States has become a fast-food, junk-food society that has led to the degradation of healthy eating habits. Obesity has risen to epidemic levels among children, adolescents, and adults. If current trends continue, obesity stands to replace cigarette smoking as the number one non-disease killer in this country. One of the primary causes of overweight problems in children and adolescents is poor eating habits. Poor eating habits are directly linked to several health problems, including heart disease, hypertension, high cholesterol, diabetes, and some cancers.

Our goal at Fresh Baby is to help you give your baby the very best start in life by providing you with all the information and products you need to prepare nutritious, fresh food and to teach your children healthy eating habits. We'd like to thank you for trying our product and doing what is best for your baby! We hope you enjoy Fresh Baby's Fresh Start Kit. Above all,

HAVE FUN!

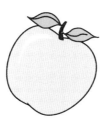

Feeding Memories and Fun

First Meal

Photo of my
first meal

My first solid food: _____
My first juice: _____

My favorite meals:

Breakfast: _____
_____

Lunch: _____
_____

Dinner: _____
_____

Snack: _____

I drank from a cup at: _____

I started feeding myself at: _____

I spit out my food on: _____

I threw my food on: _____

Photo of
me eating

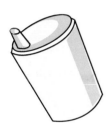

Food Reviews

👍 Yummy   Yucky 👎

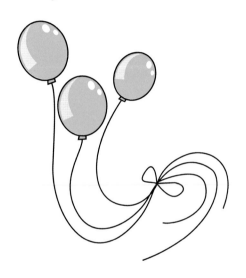

First Holiday

Photo of
my first holiday

My first holiday: _____
Age: _____
Menu: _____
_____
_____
Comments: _____
_____

First Birthday

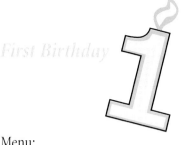

Menu:

Comments:

Photo of
my first birthday

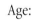
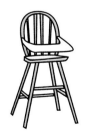

My first restaraunt:

Age:

Menu:

Comments:

Healthy Eating Habits

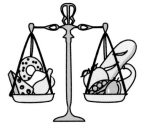

Introducing solid food usually begins at 4-6 months of age and does not have a tremendous nutritional impact. It's considered a supplement to breast milk or infant formula, which remains the primary source of nutrition until your baby is about 12 months old. So even if you don't know much about nutrition and healthy eating habits, you have about 6-8 months to begin learning and there is no better way than to make baby food at home. If you already have healthy eating habits, most likely you will pass them on to your children, and there's no better time to start than at the very beginning of their lives.

Having healthy eating habits does not mean dieting. Unless your baby's diet is under the supervision of a health care provider, it is not necessary to count calories or choose low-fat or non-fat foods. Ensuring healthy eating habits for babies is simply a matter of providing them with a varied diet and limiting the consumption of most processed foods.

Tips for encouraging healthy eating habits

1 **Take your baby to the store or local farm stands.** Begin introducing your baby to different fruits and vegetables. Teach him the names of different types of produce. Talk to him about the colors of each one and how to tell if they are ripe.

2 **Talk positively about vegetables and fruits.** Let your baby know what he is eating when you are feeding him, what vitamins and minerals he is getting, and how important nutrients are for growing bigger and stronger.

3 Be a good role model. Babies learn through mimicking you and others around them. If you talk negatively about fruits and vegetables or don't eat them much yourself, your baby will have a tough time accepting them. Remember, your baby will respond to what you like.

4 Encourage drinking water. Water aids in digestion, regulates body temperature, delivers nutrients to cells, and carries waste away. As your baby is introduced to solid food, the need for water is greater. Offer your baby 2-4 ounces of water at each meal.

5 Don't give up. Babies' tastes change on a daily basis. Just because your baby spit out peas one day does not mean he doesn't like them. Unless he has demonstrated an allergic reaction, try the food again in a couple days—you may be pleasantly surprised.

6 Offer variety to ensure a balanced diet. All foods contain different vitamins, minerals, and nutrients. Eating a variety of foods will naturally lead to a balanced diet. When your baby first starts eating, quantity is not as important as variety.

7 Don't be in a rush. Many babies are slow eaters, and this is a good habit to encourage. Many of us do not plan enough time to eat meals and often finding ourselves shoveling food in—this is one of the worst eating habits that you can teach your baby. Instead, allow plenty of time for meals so you and your baby can relax and enjoy the experience.

8 Have a feeding schedule. Establishing set times for breakfast, lunch, dinner, and snacks will help your baby learn to have three meals a day. The times at which you feed your baby will likely change with his development stages. You need to be flexible about times and pay attention to the signals he is giving you.

9 Never force babies to eat or finish all their food. Your baby will eat when he is hungry. And he will eat the types of food his body needs most. During meals allow him to eat as much or little as he wants.

10 Make mealtimes a family event. Whenever it is practical, the whole family should eat together. This will encourage your baby to interact with others at mealtime and to begin experiencing a sense of social interaction.

Preparing for the toddler phase

Your child naturally learns about food and acquires eating habits gradually as he grows older. Learning to eat is a process, like sleeping, potty training, or any other developmental skill. Each phase builds upon the previous one. The Fresh Start Kit is designed to support you through the first phase—Introducing Solid Foods. During these important 8-10 months your baby will slowly be introduced to, and learn to master, a variety of different tastes, textures, and smells.

The second developmental phase begins when your baby becomes a toddler. In terms of feeding, your baby reaches the toddler phase when breast feeding or formula feeding stops or decreases significantly. The nutritional aspect of solid food becomes much more important. While you still have several months until your family reaches this phase, here are some ways to begin preparing for it.

Become familiar with the food pyramid.

The USDA developed the food pyramid in 1992. Many of us learned about the four food groups—these are old ideas, and the pyramid is a much more intuitive way to think about eating. Its shape is designed to suggest the relative daily intake of each food category. The categories are:

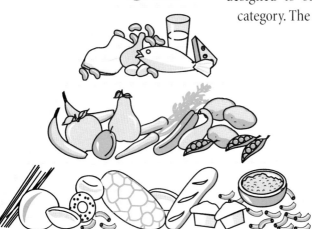

- o **Level 1**: Grains
- o **Level 2**: Fresh Produce: Fruits and Vegetables
- o **Level 3**: Proteins—Dairy and Meat and other proteins
- o **Level 4**: Fats and Sweets

While the recommended number of servings in each of these categories seems high, the actual amount per serving is really quite small. Here are some examples of serving sizes recommended by the American Academy of Pediatrics for children 1 to 3 years old.

Food Group	Serving Size
Grains 6-11 servings per day	Bread, ½ slice
	Cereal, rice, pasta, ¼ cup cooked
	Cereal, dry, ⅓ cup
	Crackers, 2-3
Vegetables 2-3 servings per day	Vegetables, cooked, ¼ cup
Fruits 2-3 servings per day	Fruit, cooked or canned, ¼ cup
	Fruit, fresh, ½ piece
	Juice, ¼ cup
Dairy 2-3 servings per day	Milk, ½ cup
	Cheese, ½ ounce
	Yogurt, ⅓ cup
Meats and other proteins 2-4 servings per day	Meat, fish, poultry,
	tofu, 1 ounce (two 1-inch cubes)
	Beans, diced and cooked, ¼ cup
	Egg, ½

Read nutrition labels on foods.

You don't have to become a nutritionist to make sure your child acquires healthy eating habits. However, it is important to understand the basics of nutrition, and the Nutrition Facts labels on most packaged foods help out a great deal. Take notice of the serving size as it relates to the rest of the information, especially sugar, sodium, and fat content. Some products may appear nutritious until you realize that the information is based on a serving size so small that you would need to multiply it by 10 to make a realistic serving size for you or your children.

Read ingredients labels on packaged foods.

You may be surprised to learn what is in some of your favorite foods. In fact, you may read the whole list and still not really know what is in these products. Ingredients are listed on the package from the highest weight by volume to the lowest. Some products, especially organic and all-natural products, are quite nutritious and contain few or no additives or preservatives. As a general rule, buy products that have common ingredients found in your kitchen.

Avoid adding sugar and fat to your family's diet.

Both sugar and fat are present naturally in many foods—and in quantities that are most likely sufficient to provide an adequate intake of this category. A few things to note:

- Eggs, whole-milk dairy products, and avocados are high in saturated fats, but they contain many other nutritional benefits and are considered good foods for your growing child.
- Processed foods often contain hydrogenated oils, which are commonly used to improve the shelf life of products and to allow fast-food restaurants to reuse deep-frying oils. Hydrogenated oils contain transfatty acids that are linked to heart disease and are known carcinogens.
- Sugary foods, such as candy, soda, and commercially baked goods, do not provide anything that your child needs for growth.

Develop alternatives to junk food.

Instead of stocking the pantry and freezer with potato chips, candy, cake, soda, cookies, and ice cream, make or buy healthier snacks for the whole family. Try these alternatives:

- Whole-grain crackers
- Rice cakes and puffed rice cereals
- Baked snack chips (there many new varieties that use vegetables instead of potatoes)
- Juice coolers made with sparkling water and 100% fruit juice
- Smoothies made with fresh fruit, yogurt, or sorbet
- Dried fruits, nuts, and seeds—apricots, raisins, cherries, cranberries, plums, almonds, pecans, walnuts, and sunflower and pumpkins seeds
- Cookies made from real fruit or fruit juice

Benefits of Home-Prepared Baby Food

resh Baby's baby food preparation system has so many benefits, including:

- o Increased nutritional value
- o Elimination of additives
- o Improved freshness
- o Additional variety
- o Enhanced control
- o Lower costs

Increased nutritional value

Vitamins and other nutrients are critically important to your baby. For the next three years, he will experience rapid growth and development. It is essential that he be fed a healthy and nutritious diet in order to maximize his growth and development process.

Processed baby foods have added water, sugars, and starchy fillers. While these products are not nutritionally bad for your baby, their use in baby food greatly dilutes the nutrient content of the actual foods. You can see the difference between the products of various food manufacturers; one brand of sweet potatoes may have a different nutritional value than another. This is caused by dilution.

To make matters even worse, processed baby foods are cooked at extremely high temperatures to kill all bacteria so they can be stored in jars at room temperature. Bacteria are not the only things that are eliminated in this process: Vitamins and nutrients are also destroyed. Many baby food manufacturers compensate for the loss of vitamins by adding them back in after the food is processed.

Elimination of additives

Processed baby foods contain trace amounts of chemicals, including pesticides, herbicides, and fungicides. Although the FDA has approved these chemicals, you may choose not to feed your baby products containing them. Buying certified organic produce (fresh or frozen) and preparing food at home using the Fresh Baby system eliminates agricultural chemicals from your baby's diet.

Improved freshness

Did you know that baby food could be up to three years old when you buy it on the grocery store shelf? And if you have ever opened a jar of processed baby food and taken a bite, you will certainly know what is meant by taste or lack thereof. Processed baby food also does not have much smell or color. Most of these attributes are removed in the manufacturing process—with the ultimate benefit being a shelf life of two to three years.

Shelf life is a great benefit to food manufacturers and retailers—not to you or your baby. While your baby does not have the refined palate of an adult, he does respond to taste, color, and smell. With the enormous availability of fresh and even frozen produce in grocery stores and the ease and convenience of home baby food preparation, there really is no reason he needs to be deprived of colorful, tasty, great-smelling baby food. Serving fresh food from the very beginning will help him be more open to tasting new flavors and types of food.

Additional variety

Processed baby food is developed for the mass market and, as a result, is limited in variety. Variety is key to a balanced diet, which is a core component of healthy and nutritious eating. With the amount of choice that is available in the produce and frozen-food sections of grocery stores with Fresh Baby, there is no reason why your baby should be limited by what food manufacturers consider the most popular foods. What's more, preparing baby food at home enables you to add herbs and combine flavors so that his mealtime is a gourmet experience.

Enhanced control

As a parent, you want to understand and trust the ingredients in your baby's diet. Similarly, you want assurance concerning the purity, safety, quality, and consistency of such ingredients. Preparing baby food at home with the Fresh Baby system provides you with control of your baby's diet and knowledge of exactly what goes into your baby's food. The more involvement you have with what you are feeding your baby, the more likely you are to nurture healthy eating habits.

Lower costs

Why pay for the marketing, advertising, and packaging associated with processed baby food that could be up to three years older than your baby? Processed baby foods are expensive. The average baby in the United States will consume 600 jars of baby food. Parents who use processed baby food spend an average of $300 or more on baby food during their infant's first year of life.

Home preparation of baby food using the Fresh Baby system is extremely cost-effective, as foods may be purchased either in season or on sale. On average, baby food prepared at home can cost as little as $55 in the first year.

Introducing Solid Foods

At Fresh Baby we believe in what is best for babies and setting the stage for healthy eating habits and nutrition. The introduction to solid foods is a very important step in your baby's development and well-being. Preparing baby food at home is a great way to ensure that your baby is getting the best in quality, nutrition, and taste.

The American Acadcmy of Pediatrics (AAP) recommends the introduction of solid food between 4 and 6 months of age. At this time, your baby's swallowing reflexes and digestive system have developed to the point where they can accept non-liquid foods. If you think your baby is ready to start solid foods, consult with your baby's health care provider. We encourage you to follow the advice of your baby's health care provider as well regarding feeding and nutrition. Your baby's health care provider is the expert who is familiar with you and your baby. He or she also receives the most current health and nutritional information.

Normally, a vitamin-fortified single-grain cereal is the best choice for your baby's very first solid food. It is prepared using either breast milk or formula to develop a thick liquid consistency. Rice, barley, and oat are the most common flavors. Rice is the most commonly recommended cereal to begin with as it is well tolerated by most infants. Once cereals have been tackled and your baby has been successful in tolerating them, you are ready to move on and the fun can begin!

Fruits and Vegetables—one at a time

When starting to introduce solid food, it is very important to be aware of any allergic reactions your baby may have to the foods you are feeding him. Go slow! There is really no reason to rush. Prepare and feed only one food to your baby for 3-4 days. Record any allergic reactions on the specific food recipe page in this Cworkbook. Once you are certain there are no complications, move on to a new food.

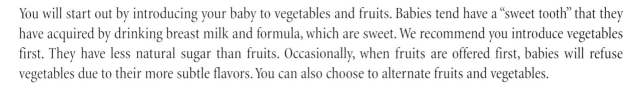

You will start out by introducing your baby to vegetables and fruits. Babies tend have a "sweet tooth" that they have acquired by drinking breast milk and formula, which are sweet. We recommend you introduce vegetables first. They have less natural sugar than fruits. Occasionally, when fruits are offered first, babies will refuse vegetables due to their more subtle flavors. You can also choose to alternate fruits and vegetables.

Food allergies

Any family history of food allergies should be discussed with your health care provider prior to introducing solid food to your baby. Once you get the go-ahead and start feeding your baby foods one at a time, watch for any changes in him. Food allergies or food intolerance can occur even if there is no family history of such.

Some common symptoms of food allergies/intolerance include:
- Rashes, especially on the face
- Diaper rash
- Hives
- Runny nose, watery eyes, or sneezing
- Diarrhea, gas, or vomiting
- Irritability
- Temperament changes
- Puffy eyes
- Nasal congestion

If you notice any of these symptoms or any other sudden, unexplained changes, notify your health care provider immediately. If a food allergy is diagnosed or suspected, make a note on the recipe page for the specific food in this book and make sure it is documented in your baby's health chart with your health care provider.

One way to prevent food allergies is not to introduce commonly allergenic food until later in your baby's life. Common allergy-producing foods include:

- Berries
- Chocolate
- Citrus fruits
- Cow's milk
- Eggs
- Fish and shellfish
- Peanuts
- Soy
- Tomatoes

If you would like to introduce these foods prior to 12 months, you should consult your health care provider and follow his or her advice.

It is not uncommon for babies to have allergic reactions to food additives, coloring agents, and preservatives commonly used in processed foods. These include ingredients such as monosodium glutamate (MSG), sulfites, nitrates, benzoates, and tartarzine. We recommend avoiding the introduction of any processed foods until your baby is at least 12 months old.

Fortunately, most allergic reactions in babies are temporary and the culprit foods can usually be reintroduced when the baby is a little older. Talk to your health care provider about your baby's reaction and consult with them on reintroducing these foods.

Herbs, spices, and natural flavors

Herbs, spices, and natural flavors are a great way to enhance the flavor and add to the variety of food without using salt or sugar. For each recipe in this book, we offer specific suggestions on the use of different herbs, spices, and natural flavors. Here are some general guidelines for introducing enhancements.

- Wait until your baby is about 8-10 months of age. His digestive system should be mature enough to handle the digestion of herbs and spices.
- Add herbs and spices only to foods that you have previously fed to your baby. Remember the "One at a Time" rule to ensure that any food allergies are detected early.
- Introduce herbs and spices sparingly at first. Your baby's palate is much more sensitive than yours, so a little goes a long way.
- If you see any signs of an allergic reaction, discontinue use of the particular herb or spice and follow our guidelines for documenting it and notifying your health care provider.

Common herbs and spices include:
- Cinnamon
- Clove
- Dill
- Ginger
- Mint
- Nutmeg
- Oregano
- Parsley

Common natural flavors include:
- Garlic
- Lemon and orange zest
- Onion
- Vanilla extract

Foods not recommended for babies

There are many foods that are not good for babies before 12 months of age.

- Honey and corn syrup should be avoided until your baby is at least 12 months old. They contain bacterial spores that can cause a form of botulism.
- Some foods are dangerous due to your baby's lack of teeth and lack of mouth/tongue coordination; offering these too early can result in choking. These foods include nuts (other than finely ground), peanut butter, caramel candy, gum, whole grapes, raw hard fruits and vegetables, chunks of meat, pieces of bacon, hot dogs, sunflower seeds, raisins, popcorn, potato or corn chips, and hard candy.
- Foods high in nitrates can cause anemia and should not be included in your child's diet until the age of 8 months. Nitrate-rich vegetables include beets, carrots, spinach, and collard greens. Meats that contain nitrates include hot dogs, cured ham, bacon, bologna, and salami.
- Avoid foods high in salt, sugar, and caffeine altogether or carefully monitor them. In most cases, foods containing high amounts of salt, sugar, or caffeine usually do not contain many vitamins and minerals. Stay away from them.

Juice

The American Academy of Pediatrics recommends waiting until your baby is 8 months old or drinking from a cup before introducing fruit juice. Follow the same rule as you do when introducing food: Juices should be tried one at a time. Use only 100 percent real juices, avoid juices that contain high fructose corn syrup or other additives, and start with only single-flavor juices, not combinations of juices. Fruit juice should be diluted with water (50/50). Limit servings to 4 ounces (½ cup). If your baby is under 12 months old, do not feed him unpasteurized fruit juice such as apple cider. These can contain disease-causing bacteria.

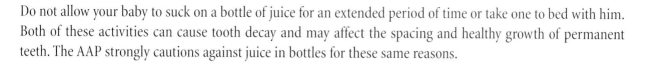

Do not allow your baby to suck on a bottle of juice for an extended period of time or take one to bed with him. Both of these activities can cause tooth decay and may affect the spacing and healthy growth of permanent teeth. The AAP strongly cautions against juice in bottles for these same reasons.

Do not make the mistake of offering your baby unlimited amounts of fruit juice. Large amounts of juice will lessen his appetite at mealtime and can also cause cramping and diarrhea. Water is an excellent substitute for juice. It quenches thirst better than juice and helps to establish a good eating habit for later in life.

Mealtime: tips on feeding

Food can be served at room temperature or slightly heated. If you use a microwave to warm food, thoroughly stir the food to eliminate any hot spots and test the temperature prior to serving. Use a small spoon with a shallow plastic bowl. The rubber-tipped baby spoons are great for first-time eaters. When introducing solid foods, be sure to offer 2-4 ounces of water at each meal. Your baby needs additional water at intervals to aid in his digestion process. The AAP recommends that babies be offered water as part of each meal, which will allow your baby to fulfill his fluid needs without consuming additional calories.

When you first start feeding your baby, plan on sitting with him and offering food for about 20 minutes per meal. Sometimes he will eat a lot, sometimes only a little. Don't panic, this is normal. Eventually your baby will let you know when he is done—telltale signs include:

- Pushing the spoon away from his mouth
- Hitting at the spoon
- Playing with his food
- Spitting food out
- Turning his head away

It is not necessary for your baby to finish his meals. The "clean plate" club is out, and forced feeding could lead to poor eating habits later in life.

Choking can occur when your baby is introduced to solid foods, so it is vital to know what to do. The American

Red Cross offers courses in infant first aid and CPR. We strongly encourage all parents and caregivers to take a course. You can find out more about this course by visiting the American Red Cross web site (http://www.americanredcross.org) or by calling the local Red Cross office in your area.

Take these preventative measures to protect your baby from choking hazards:
- Always supervise him while eating.
- Feed him while in a chair or sitting down.
- Do not allow him to crawl or walk around while eating.
- Avoid foods that are likely to cause choking (see "Foods not recommended for babies").

First Foods by Age

Age (m)	Grains	Vegetables	Fruit	Meat & Proteins	Dairy Products
4-6	Vitamin-fortified cereal—rice, barley, oat	Acorn squash, Butternut squash, Peas, Sweet potato	Apples, Banana, Pears	None	None
6-8	Same as above	Pumpkin, Yellow squash, Zucchini	Apricots, Avocado, Nectarines, Peaches, Plums	Chicken, Tofu, Turkey	Plain yogurt
8-10	Vitamin-fortified cereal—mixed, Graham crackers, Low-salt crackers, Cheerios	Asparagus, Carrots, Broccoli, Green beans, Cauliflower, Snow peas, Spinach, Sugar snap peas, White potato	Kiwi, Grapes (quartered), Mango, Papaya	Lean beef, Beans—pinto, black, white, navy, Nuts—almonds, pecans, walnuts, Seeds—sunflower, sesame	Cream cheese, Cottage cheese, Ricotta cheese
10-12	Egg-free pasta, Rice	Artichokes, Beets, Corn, Cucumber, Eggplant	Berries, Cherries, Dates, Cantaloupe, Citrus fruits, Coconut milk, Pineapple, Prunes	Lamb, Liver, Egg yolks (fully cooked)	Semi-hard cheeses (Cheddar, Swiss, Monterey Jack, Munster, Gouda)

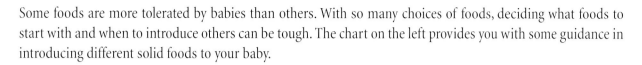

Some foods are more tolerated by babies than others. With so many choices of foods, deciding what foods to start with and when to introduce others can be tough. The chart on the left provides you with some guidance in introducing different solid foods to your baby.

Finger foods

Between 7 and 8 months you can introduce finger foods to encourage your baby to begin self-feeding. Finger foods are just as simple to make as other baby food. Simply cut up fruits or vegetables into cubes or spears, cook them in the microwave, and freeze them in your Fresh Baby trays or plastic freezer bags. When using plastic freezer bags, place small amounts in the bag and freeze them completely flat with food spread throughout the bag. The food in the bag will freeze into small chunks that will allow you to use small amounts at a time.

Examples of finger foods that can be served raw are bananas, avocados, and semi-hard cheeses. Examples of cooked finger foods are apples, pears, whole asparagus spears, carrots, zucchini or yellow squash, broccoli, whole green beans, and anything else you can think of. Use your imagination!

Tip for teething: Frozen finger foods are a great way to soothe your baby's teething pain, and they are nutritious, too.

How much is enough?

When you begin the introduction of solid foods, quantity is not as important as variety. Don't despair if your baby is eating only a few spoonfuls of food at the beginning. This is completely normal. Over the course of several months, your baby will begin to eat more solid food. By the time he reaches 12-18 months, his

Food	Servings
Whole milk	16 to 24 ounces
Fruits and vegetables	4 to 8 tablespoons
Breads and cereals	4 servings (a serving equals ¼ slice of bread or 2 tablespoons of rice, potatoes, pasta, etc.)
Meat, poultry, fish, eggs	2 servings each (about ½ ounce or 1 tablespoon)

diet will become a combination of breast milk/formula/whole milk and solid foods. The American Academy of Pediatrics provides the above guidelines for a baby's minimum daily food intake at about 12-18 months.

Dietary Essentials for Your Baby's Diet

The foods your child eats are necessary for proper functioning and development. These are especially important to babies, since they are still growing and developing. Dietary essentials are fats, carbohydrates, proteins, and vitamins and minerals.

Fats

Fats are a very important part of your baby's diet. They provide vitamins A, D, E, K, and linoleic acid, which prevent skin problems and growth retardation. According to the American Academy of Pediatrics, the calorie intake of your baby's diet should be 50 percent from fat, and nutrition experts recommend gradually decreasing this amount to 33 percent after the age of 2 years. Babies and children need significantly more fat than adults do. Polyunsaturated fats are essential to good health; they are also necessary for the absorption of the fat-soluble vitamins.

Carbohydrates

Carbohydrates are used primarily as a source of energy. They appear in the form of starches and sugars. Your baby needs extra energy to keep warm and assist his body in growing. Carbohydrates help the body use fat and protein and help keep the liver healthy. Complex carbohydrates, unlike refined carbohydrates (sugars such as table sugar, honey, and syrups), provide increased stamina. Although many adults consider carbohydrates fattening, carbohydrates allow your baby's system to use them first for energy, thereby enabling protein to be used for tissue and muscle growth.

Proteins

Proteins are essential for cell growth, muscle and tissue repair, reproduction, and protection against infection. For the most part, your baby's protein needs are being met for the first 12 months by breast milk or formula. Additional protein intake in your baby's diet does become essential after the first year.

Vitamins

Vitamins are categorized as fat-soluble or water-soluble. Fat-soluble vitamins include A, D, E, and K. Water soluble vitamins include the B-complex group and C. Fat-soluble vitamins can be stored for later use by the body. Water-soluble vitamins are excreted in the urine and, therefore, must be eaten daily in order to supply the body constantly. The body uses vitamins for many different functions—from cell development to immunity and nervous-system maintenance.

Minerals

Minerals, like vitamins, are also very important to your baby's diet, because his body needs them to grow, develop, and maintain health. Minerals are obtained the same way you get vitamins: from food. The body uses minerals to perform many different functions—from building strong bones to transmitting nerve impulses. Some minerals are even used to make hormones or maintain a normal heart beat.

There are two kinds of minerals: macro-minerals and trace minerals. Macro means "large" in Greek (and your body needs larger amounts of macro-minerals than trace minerals). The macro-mineral group is made up of calcium, phosphorous, magnesium, sodium, potassium, chloride, and sulfur.

A trace of something means that your baby needs only a little of it. So even though your baby needs trace minerals, he needs just a tiny bit of each one. Scientists aren't even sure how much of these minerals you need each day! The trace mineral crowd includes iron, manganese, copper, iodine, zinc, cobalt, fluoride, and selenium.

Health benefits of vitamins and minerals

Everyone has heard of vitamins and minerals, but what can they really do for our health? The chart below explains why we need them and what each of them does.

Vitamin	Health Benefit
Vitamin A	Important for good vision, prevents night blindness. Also affects immunity, reproduction, and the growth and maintenance of cells of the skin, gastrointestinal tract, and other mucous membranes. Promotes healthy skin, hair, and nails
Vitamin B$_1$ or Thiamin	Important for producing energy from carbohydrates and for proper nerve function
Vitamin B$_2$ or Riboflavin	Contributes to energy production
Vitamin B$_3$ or Niacin	Contributes to energy production. Important for health of skin, digestive tract, and nervous system
Biotin	Contributes to energy production and metabolism of proteins, fats, and carbohydrates
Pantothenic Acid	Contributes to energy production
Vitamin B$_6$	Helps the body make red blood cells, converts tryptophan to niacin, and contributes to immunity and nervous system function. Used in metabolism of proteins and fats
Folic Acid	Critical for all cell functions, since folic acid helps make DNA and RNA. May protect against heart disease by lowering homocysteine levels. In pregnant women, lowers risk of neural tube defects in the baby
Vitamin B$_{12}$	Important for proper nerve function. Works with folic acid, converting it to an active form. Helps make red blood cells and helps metabolize proteins and fats
Vitamin C	Important for immune function. Acts as an antioxidant to keep the body healthy. Strengthens blood vessels and capillary walls, makes collagen and connective tissue that hold muscles and bones
Vitamin D	Increases absorption of calcium and phosphorus, which leads to stronger bones and teeth
Vitamin E	Acts as an antioxidant, reducing the risks of cancer and heart disease; contributes to good immunity. Protects body tissues, including eyes, skin, and liver. Protects lungs from being damaged by polluted air. Necessary for normal clotting of blood
Vitamin K	Makes proteins that allow the blood to clot

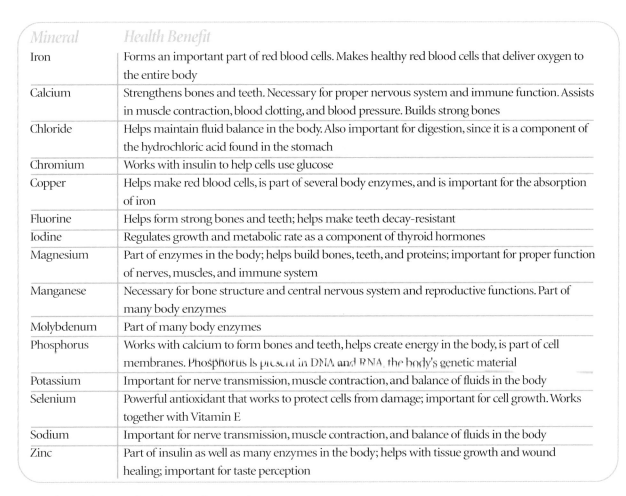

Mineral	Health Benefit
Iron	Forms an important part of red blood cells. Makes healthy red blood cells that deliver oxygen to the entire body
Calcium	Strengthens bones and teeth. Necessary for proper nervous system and immune function. Assists in muscle contraction, blood clotting, and blood pressure. Builds strong bones
Chloride	Helps maintain fluid balance in the body. Also important for digestion, since it is a component of the hydrochloric acid found in the stomach
Chromium	Works with insulin to help cells use glucose
Copper	Helps make red blood cells, is part of several body enzymes, and is important for the absorption of iron
Fluorine	Helps form strong bones and teeth; helps make teeth decay-resistant
Iodine	Regulates growth and metabolic rate as a component of thyroid hormones
Magnesium	Part of enzymes in the body; helps build bones, teeth, and proteins; important for proper function of nerves, muscles, and immune system
Manganese	Necessary for bone structure and central nervous system and reproductive functions. Part of many body enzymes
Molybdenum	Part of many body enzymes
Phosphorus	Works with calcium to form bones and teeth, helps create energy in the body, is part of cell membranes. Phosphorus is present in DNA and RNA, the body's genetic material
Potassium	Important for nerve transmission, muscle contraction, and balance of fluids in the body
Selenium	Powerful antioxidant that works to protect cells from damage; important for cell growth. Works together with Vitamin E
Sodium	Important for nerve transmission, muscle contraction, and balance of fluids in the body
Zinc	Part of insulin as well as many enzymes in the body; helps with tissue growth and wound healing; important for taste perception

Vitamin and mineral supplements

There are a variety of liquid vitamin and mineral supplements available for babies. Although it can depend on where you live and the type of water your baby is consuming, the AAP does recommend a fluoride-containing supplement to babies after 6 months of age. Before giving your baby any vitamin or mineral supplements, consult your health care provider for advice.

Making and Serving Fresh Baby Food

The recipe section of this book provides you with detailed instructions on the preparation of each food that is featured. This section also offers general advice and guidance in making and serving baby food.

Selecting produce

Selecting fresh produce is important for nutrition, texture, and flavor. Each Fresh Baby recipe contains tips on how to determine ripeness of the main fruit or vegetable. The following are some general pointers on shopping for fresh produce.

- Choose fresh-looking fruits and vegetables that are not bruised, shriveled, moldy, or slimy.
- Don't buy anything that smells bad.
- Don't buy packaged vegetables that have a lot of liquid in the bag or that look slimy. Some fruits, such as fresh-cut pineapple, will have liquid in the bag, and that's okay.
- Buy only what you need because most fruits and vegetables are not "stock-up" items. Some, such as apples and potatoes, can be stored at home, but most items should be used within a few days.
- Handle produce carefully at the store. Keep produce on top in your shopping cart (heavy items on top will bruise fruits and vegetables, and raw meat products might drip juices on them).
- Set produce gently on the checkout belt so it doesn't bruise. Some items that may seem hardy, such as cauliflower, actually are very delicate and bruise easily.
- Remember to wash produce just before you use it, not when you put it away.

Cooking the Fresh Baby Way

It is very easy and quick to prepare baby food at home. Each food included in this Cworkbook has a specific recipe. This section introduces you to the basic concept.

Step 1: **Prep**—Depending on the type of baby food you are preparing, you will need to wash, chop, and peel the fruits and vegetables. You should not use detergent or bleach when washing fruits and vegetables because these chemicals can leave a residue that will be absorbed by porous food like produce. If you are using frozen produce, thaw and simply open the package.

Step 2: **Cook**—Cook the food in the microwave or use the stovetop method of steaming with natural herbs or spices. All preparation times in this book are based on the microwave method. We recommend cooking in the microwave for several reasons:
- Saves time because food cooks faster
- Retains more nutrients because food is cooked faster with little to no water
- Easier cleanup

Step 3: **Puree**—Pour the food and cooking juices into a food processor or a blender and puree. This is the most important step in making your baby food. Food consistency is created during this step. You want your baby to have food that is soft and velvety in texture. You may need to add a little water to some foods to get the right consistency. Although water will slightly dilute the food's nutritional value, the difference is not significant enough to worry about. After 8 months, you can use unsweetened, 100% fruit juice, vegetable broth, or chicken stock (homemade with no salt or, if using canned stock, with reduced sodium) instead of water.

Step 4: **Pour**—Pour the food into the Fresh Baby freezer trays and freeze. The Fresh Baby freezer trays have covers to keep freezer odor out.

Step 5: **Freeze**—Place the trays in the freezer for 8-10 hours or overnight. Remove the baby food cubes from the freezer trays and store the cubes in the freezer for up to two months. You may have to run a little hot water on the trays to make removal of food cubes easy. You can use plastic freezer storage bags or stackable plastic containers to store food. Make sure that you label all food with the type of food and the date it was prepared.

Serving the Fresh Baby Way

Serving your baby food with the Fresh Baby food cube system is simple and fast. There is also plenty of room for creativity to make your baby's mealtime a gourmet experience.

Thawing baby food cubes

It is easy to get ready for a meal. Simply select baby food cubes from the freezer and place them in a dish. You can use one of these methods for thawing:

- *Microwave:* Thawing food in the microwave is the fastest approach. Simply place a microwave-safe dish containing food cubes in the microwave and defrost them. You will find that some foods defrost faster than others do. Defrosting two dishes of food at once may take a little longer.
- *Refrigerator:* Thawing food in the refrigerator is the easiest but requires planning ahead. Simply place a covered dish containing food cubes in the refrigerator. In about 3-4 hours they will thaw. You can warm them (if desired) in the microwave.

* *Note:* Microwaves create hot spots in food. When using a microwave to thaw or warm baby food, stir the food well before serving. Always check the temperature of the food before serving. Food that is too hot to eat can be cooled quickly by placing it in the freezer for a few seconds.

Thinning and thickening baby food

Most baby food should have a soft, velvety consistency (if you are just starting to feed your baby solid food, thinner is better than thicker).

Mixing different foods together can help achieve the right consistency. For example, zucchini tends to

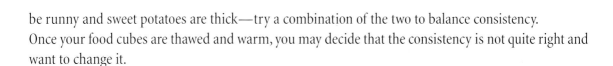

be runny and sweet potatoes are thick—try a combination of the two to balance consistency. Once your food cubes are thawed and warm, you may decide that the consistency is not quite right and want to change it.

Thickeners: The most nutritious way to thicken baby food is to add vitamin-fortified dry cereal to it. This also has the extra benefit of adding more vitamins to your baby's meal. Mashed banana and yogurt are also great thickeners and appeal to many babies.

Thinners: The most nutritious way to thin baby food is to add breast milk or formula. Your baby is familiar with the taste of either breast milk or formula and it provides a good vitamin supplement to a baby's meal. For older babies, 100% real juice or soup stock (vegetable or chicken) can be used to thin food.

Creating medleys

Once your baby has been introduced to a variety of foods using the "one at a time" method, you can begin making meals more interesting and introduce an array of tastes to your baby. Each Fresh Baby frozen food cube is a one-ounce serving (about 1 Tablespoon). By mixing together different cubes and other foods, like grains, dairy products, and proteins, you can create tasty medleys at each meal. For each recipe included in this book, we offer specific medley combinations to try. Here are some examples:

- Peas and sweet potatoes
- Green beans and white potatoes
- Broccoli, cauliflower, and melted cheese
- Butternut squash, corn, and tofu
- Peaches, pears, rice cereal, and almonds
- Raspberries, apples, yogurt, and walnuts

Tip: Many baby food manufacturers make medleys or "meals in a jar." Read the labels to get ideas on what to serve at home for your baby.

Kitchen Tools

Most of the tools you need to prepare baby food are already in your kitchen or included in your Fresh Baby Fresh Start Kit. We strongly encourage reviewing the video included in your Fresh Start Kit. This video provides a demonstration of the process of making baby food. In addition to this Cworkbook, here is what you will need:

Step 1: **Prep tools**

If you have decided to use frozen produce, this step is eliminated. For fresh produce, you will need:

- Cutting board—Either wood or plastic will do. The cutting board should always be washed with soap and hot water prior to using it
- Paring knife
- Peeler
- Spoon
- Colander or strainer (optional but helpful)

Step 2: **Cooking tools**

- Potholders/oven mitts
- Microwave-safe dish and cover (microwave method)
- Saucepan and steamer basket (stovetop method)

Step 3: **Pureeing tools**

- Blender/food processor—A food processor is your best choice. If you don't have a food processor, here is the perfect reason to buy one and learn how to use it.
- Rubber spatula or scraper

Step 4 : ***Pouring tools***
- Spatula
- Fresh Baby freezer trays with covers

Step 5 : ***Freezing tools***
- Freezer bags or freezer storage containers
- Permanent marker

Step 6 : ***Serving Tools***
- Plastic bowls (microwave-safe)
- Spoon—the long-handled, rubber-tipped ones are ideal
- Feeding bib
- Paper towels or washcloth for cleanup

Safety Basics

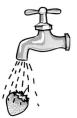

General

- All baby food should be cooked thoroughly, with the exception of bananas, tofu, and avocados. Check with your health care provider for guidance on when to introduce raw foods.
- Clean all utensils and work surfaces before preparing baby food. Any equipment that was previously used to handle raw foods (especially chicken, meat, and eggs) should be washed thoroughly with dish detergent and hot water.
- Wash your hands before beginning to make baby food and make sure your hands are clean throughout the process.
- Keep hot foods hot and cold foods cold to prevent bacteria growth. Don't let prepared baby food sit at room temperature more than one hour. If you get distracted and don't have time to put it in freezer trays, cover it and place it in the refrigerator until later.

Cooking

- Thoroughly wash all fruits and vegetables, even if you are using organic produce.
- Follow the cooking time and standing time directions. All stoves and microwaves vary slightly in temperature and power. Check to make sure the food you are preparing is cooked. If you can easily pierce the food with a fork, it is done.
- Use microwave-safe cookware and wraps when cooking food in the microwave.
- Wrap or cover foods completely to trap steam when cooking.

Storage

- Carefully label and date all foods that are stored in the freezer. Baby food stored in the freezer will last two months.
- Hold any unused leftovers in the refrigerator. Defrosted baby food will last 1-2 days in the refrigerator.
- Do not save food that the baby spoon or your baby has touched.
- Discard any food that has been standing out for 2 hours.
- Do not refreeze defrosted cooked food.
- When traveling, always take baby food in an insulated cooler or tote bag.

Serving

- Test food for temperature before serving. Babies can be fed food at room temperature or slightly warmed. Baby food should never be served hot.
- Stir food to evenly distribute heat. If food is too hot to serve, place it in the freezer for a few seconds to cool it down.
- Use plastic or paper to serve food, even if you are spoon-feeding. It is highly likely that your baby will find some way to toss the dish or make you drop it.
- Use a spoon to feed your baby. The plastic or rubber-dipped spoons are best for your baby.
- Always have your baby in a sitting position when fed. Not only is it easier to feed them, but it is also a precaution against choking. You may not be able to use a high chair for the first few months of feeding. Sit your baby on your lap or in a bouncy seat or stroller.

Food Choices

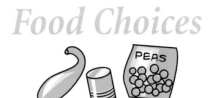

Fresh versus frozen versus canned

When it comes time to select fruits and vegetables for your baby, here are some choices to consider. As a general rule of thumb, avoid canned fruits and vegetables. Canned fruits and vegetables contain higher amounts of salt (sodium) than fresh or frozen. And many contain added sugar in the form of corn syrup, fruit juice concentrates, or fructose. One exception to this rule is tomatoes. If you want to feed tomatoes to your baby, you can choose a canned "fresh" variety and carefully read the label to ensure that you are buying just tomatoes. We also recommend using canned beans (legumes) for your baby. Canned beans are much quicker to prepare than the dried variety. Look for a low-sodium variety and rinse them for at least one minute before using.

Fresh versus frozen-nutritional value

Many people assume that because fresh produce is fresher, it automatically contains a higher nutrient value than frozen. In most cases, this is not true. The nutrient value of fresh and frozen produce is, in most cases, the same. While commercial processing does destroy some of the nutrients in the food, a number of other factors can cause even greater nutrient loss:

- Careless transportation
- Poorly designed store displays
- Improper storage at home
- Prolonged cooking
- Age of the produce

In some cases, frozen food may actually be more nutritious than fresh food. For example, if freezing occurs immediately after harvesting when nutrient content is greatest, the nutrients are preserved until the package is opened. Fresh produce, on the other hand, must travel from the farm to the store to your dinner table, which could take weeks or months and which will result in a loss of nutrients.

Here are some tips to prevent nutrient loss in the produce you purchase:

When buying frozen:

- Avoid bulk bags of fruits and vegetables that feel like a solid brick. What's inside should move about freely.
- Avoid selecting boxed frozen fruits or vegetables with colored stains or leaking liquid. These are all signs that thawing and refreezing have taken place, causing a loss of quality, and possibly of nutrients.

When buying fresh:

- Plan on using it immediately. Even if you refrigerate it, produce will continue to lose half or more of some of its vitamins within one to two weeks.
- Keep the peels on, as this also helps to preserve nutrients.

When cooking vegetables to preserve nutrient content, use very little water. The following methods are in order of best to worst:
- **Best:** microwave with little or no water; covered to trap steam
- **Second-best approach:** steaming with a small amount of water
- **Worst:** boiling in lots of water

Fresh versus frozen—other considerations

There are benefits to both types of produce for you and your baby. Consider the following:
- Fresh is most often cheaper than frozen. In almost all cases, frozen foods will be more expensive than the same fresh variety.

- Seasonal produce is available year-round frozen. A number of different fruits and vegetables are available fresh for very short periods during the year. These include cherries, strawberries, asparagus, artichokes, etc.
- Frozen produce saves time. Since it is ready to cook, there is little to no preparation time. It can be a big time-saver for parents.
- Some produce is difficult to find fresh.

Organic versus commercial

Today, many people believe that purchasing organic produce, both fresh and frozen, is healthier. The assumption is that pesticides, herbicides, and fungicides, which create residues on the produce, are not used in the growing process. When making this decision to purchase organic or commercially grown produce, consider the following:

- The nutrient content of organic and commercially grown produce is likely to be the same.
- Many herbicides, fungicides, and insecticides used in commercially grown crops are known to cause cancer.
- Per pound of body weight, babies consume, on average, 60 times more fruits and vegetables than adults do.
- Fresh produce is often transported long distances. In order to keep produce fresh, sulfides are used during transportation.
- Proper cleaning of fresh produce, including soaking, rinsing, and peeling, can reduce levels of residue by 30-100 percent.
- Organic produce, both fresh and frozen, is more expensive than commercially grown produce.

Fresh Baby To Go

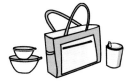

These days, families are always on the go, whether it's off to day care everyday or to visit friends and family once in a while. Here are some strategies to help you prepare for your baby's meals on the go. Start with the six golden storage rules for serving Fresh Baby away from home:

1. Frozen food cubes take 3-4 hours to thaw in the refrigerator and 1-2 hours to thaw at room temperature.
2. Frozen food cubes stay cold in an insulated bag with a freezer pack for about 8-12 hours.
3. To thaw frozen food cubes, microwave 30-40 seconds.
4. To warm thawed food cubes, microwave 5-15 seconds.
5. Never store frozen food cubes without refrigeration for over 4 hours.
6. Always test the temperature of microwaved or warmed food on your skin before serving to your baby.

Once you've got the basics, you're on your way! Tips for packing and special destinations are addressed below.

Travel tote bag

A travel tote bag is an essential item for any family on the go. Buy the Fresh Baby Travel Tote or create one yourself by purchasing a set of plastic containers with plastic lids and an insulated lunch bag. The best type of lunch bag to purchase is a sturdy canvas tote that comes with an ice pack—the type you can place in the freezer overnight. Also consider the size so it will fit easily into a diaper bag.

If you plan to be visiting friends and family frequently, consider buying a portable high chair. There are a number of them that attach to a chair or table and are very lightweight or even have a carry case. Keep it in your car so you are always prepared for an impromptu stop.

Day care

Getting meals ready for your baby's day away from home is easy. You will need a travel tote bag. Write your baby's name on the travel tote bag and the freezer pack with a permanent marker.

In the morning or before you leave for day care, select the food cubes for your baby's meal(s) from the freezer and place them in the plastic containers and seal them with the lids. If you are providing more than one meal or snack, provide the caregiver with easy instructions. For example, label each lid "Lunch," "Snack," and "Dinner" with a permanent marker.

If your day care provider has a refrigerator, there is no need to use the freezer pack. When you arrive at the facility, place the travel tote bag in the refrigerator. By the time lunch rolls around, the food will be thawed and ready to serve. If there is no refrigerator, put the food and the freezer pack in the travel tote and your baby is ready to go. If your baby likes his food warm, you may want to provide verbal instructions to your caregiver and add them in written form in the travel tote bag.

Don't forget to pack the spoon, bib, and a bottle of water for your baby's meals!

Restaurants

Going to a restaurant is great experience for the family. When deciding on where to go:
- Make reservations so you do not have to wait to be seated.
- Plan the time to have dinner or lunch according to your baby's feeding schedule.
- Call ahead to find out if the restaurant has a high chair.
- Make sure the table you sit at has adequate room for everyone, including your baby.
- Remove everything within reach of your baby—unless you want to see it on the floor.

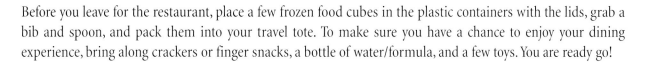

Before you leave for the restaurant, place a few frozen food cubes in the plastic containers with the lids, grab a bib and spoon, and pack them into your travel tote. To make sure you have a chance to enjoy your dining experience, bring along crackers or finger snacks, a bottle of water/formula, and a few toys. You are ready go!

Fresh Baby food cubes take about 1-2 hours to thaw. If you arrive at the restaurant and they are still frozen, ask the waiter to microwave them for 15-20 seconds. Commercial microwaves are much stronger than consumer ones, so make sure you test the temperature of the food before feeding it to your baby.

Remember that a baby's moods can be very unpredictable. All babies can have their ups and downs at restaurants; don't despair if he is not the perfect child. If your baby is acting up at the restaurant table, try a stroll around the parking lot or the block. If that doesn't work, you can always take your meal to go and enjoy a candlelit dinner with your spouse after your little one has gone to bed.

Dinner at a friend's house

When you have plans for dinner and you are bringing your baby, call a few days in advance to find out if your friends have a high chair or have access to one. If there is no high chair available, you can feed your baby in his stroller or bouncy seat. But as your baby gets older this alternative will disappear and he will want to socialize at the dinner table with everyone else.

Before leaving your home, place a few frozen food cubes in the plastic containers with the lids, grab a bib and spoon, pack them into your travel tote. To enjoy your whole dinner, bring along some crackers or finger snacks, a bottle of water/formula, and a few toys. You are ready go!

Food cubes take about 1-2 hours to thaw. When you arrive at your friend's home just place them in the refrigerator until you are ready to feed him.

Day, plane, train, or bus trips

Planning to get away for a day or going on an airplane, train, or bus and need to pack up your baby's meals? If your baby is at day care, you are already a pro. If this is the first time, it is easy to get ready for a day away from home.

Just before you are ready to leave on your trip, select the foods cubes for your baby's meal(s) and place them in the plastic containers and seal them with the lids. If you pack more than one meal or snack, label the lids of the containers "Lunch," "Snack," and "Dinner" with a permanent marker. This makes it easy to grab what you need for the meal, especially when you are feeding him in the car seat. Pack them in your travel tote bag with the freezer pack.

If you are packing for more than one meal, bring an extra bib and spoon, just in case there is no place to wash the dirty ones. Using frozen food cubes and the freezer pack will keep your food cold for about 8-12 hours— plenty of time for your trip. Some airlines, especially international carriers, will provide baby food. When making your reservations, ask about this type of meal service.

Plan the number of bottles of formula you will need. Powdered formula is the best for traveling. Measure out the amounts needed and place them in the bottles. Don't count on having access to a place to wash and clean bottles. Bring water in a separate container. When it is time for a bottle, just add the water to the bottle, shake it up, and you are ready to go. If your baby is drinking milk, buy it on the road or ask for it on the plane instead of trying to keep it cold.

If you are on the road and need a bottle or food warmed, most convenience stores and truck stops have microwaves. Or stop at a restaurant and ask the hostess to warm up the bottle/food for you. Most establishments are more than happy to help out. Airplanes do not have microwaves; the flight attendant will provide you with a bag of very hot water to warm bottles and food. Just be careful with this bag while you are holding it.

Vacations

Vacations are a terrific time to bond and introduce your little one to new things in life. While you can bring all your stuff to make baby food with you, you might consider buying jarred food for the time away. After all, Mom and Dad are on vacation, too. However, there are few things you still need to plan for your trip.

Staying at a hotel? There are so many choices available in today's hotel industry. The best type of hotel to choose will have:

- A refrigerator and microwave in the room. Even though you are not making food, once a jar of baby food has been opened, it requires refrigeration. And if your baby likes warm food and bottles, you will need to warm them up. If you don't have a microwave, you can always use the hot water method of warming.
- Buffet/Continental breakfast. Many hotels have an open area for breakfast with a flexible time period of availability. It is a comfortable way for everyone to get started in the morning—instead of having to worry about getting in the car and going to a restaurant.
- A crib for the room. Nearly ever hotel will provide a crib for your baby to sleep in. Make sure you reserve one in advance to ensure one is available when you arrive.
- One bed (queen or king) or consider a suite hotel. This will provide more room for your baby to crawl or walk around and provide more comfort for everyone.
- An elevator or a ground-floor room. You will be carrying more than you are used to and just unloading can be a chore if you have to climb a flight of stairs.

If you are flying and will have access to car at your destination or you are staying in a city, call the hotel ahead of time and ask if there is a grocery store or drug store within driving/walking distance. If there is a store close by, plan on buying disposable items (diapers, baby food, wipes, etc.) at your point of destination. It will save you a lot of agony in packing and carrying luggage. If you plan to do this, pack a few extra items, just in case of an unexpected layover or stop.

Travel item checklist

Item	Day care	Restaurant	Dinner at a home	Day, plane, train, or bus trip	Vacation
Fresh Baby Travel Tote Bag	✓	✓	✓	✓	✓
Fresh Baby frozen food cubes	✓	✓	✓	✓	
Dry snacks	✓	✓	✓	✓	✓
Dish soap				✓	✓
Bottle brush				✓	✓
Dish sponge				✓	✓
Water bottle		✓		✓	✓
Bibs	✓	✓	✓	✓	✓
Spoons	✓	✓	✓	✓	✓
Serving bowls					✓
Bottles	✓	✓	✓	✓	✓
Powdered formula				✓	✓
Vitamin-fortified cereal				✓	✓
Jars of baby food					✓
Portable high chair		✓	✓	✓	✓

he Fresh Baby system is designed to be simple and quick. Once you get started, it is more convenient than buying baby food at the store. After all, you just reach into the freezer for your baby's food.

If you spend 30 minutes per week, you can easily make enough food to feed one baby. Parents with multiples can double up the recipes to make more food at once. It will only take a little bit longer for you to prepare the food.

Here are some tips that will help you out.

- *Plan ahead*. Before you go to the grocery store, look through the freezer and take a mental inventory. Read through the recipes and select something to make. Always have a backup recipe, just in case the food you wanted to purchase is not ripe, in poor condition, unavailable, or too expensive.

- *In a REAL hurry—buy frozen.* Buying frozen food saves a lot of time—it is already washed, cleaned, and ready to cook. Washing and cleaning some foods can be the most time-consuming step in the recipe.

- *Make one or two foods at a time*. Don't worry about having a lot of variety. If you make food once a week, you build up a supply in your freezer and before you know it, you will have a great variety to choose from.

- *Pick one cooking method and stick with it*. We offer instructions for microwave and stovetop cooking. Pick one method and stick with it. This will enable you to master the technique and will result in greater efficiency.

- *Plan on 30 minutes per week*. Set aside the time to make your baby food. Pick a time when you do not have distractions. In the evening after your baby has gone to sleep is a great time. Or one parent can watch the baby while the other makes food. DON'T try to make baby food with your baby in the kitchen—it will go slower, it will be frustrating, and it could even be dangerous.

- *Use the Cworkbook*. Take notes and keep a record. Your baby's personal information will help you decide what to make and will make it easier to plan. It will also remind you of allergic reactions and when they occurred. Remember, you can reintroduce foods that your baby had allergic reactions to.

- *Learn what your baby likes and double the recipes*. Some foods will become staples in your baby's diet. Learn what they are and make twice as much. If you don't have enough Fresh Baby freezer trays for double portions, you can purchase another set on our web site (http://www.myfreshbaby.com) or freeze half the recipe overnight and store the remainder in the refrigerator and freeze it the next day.

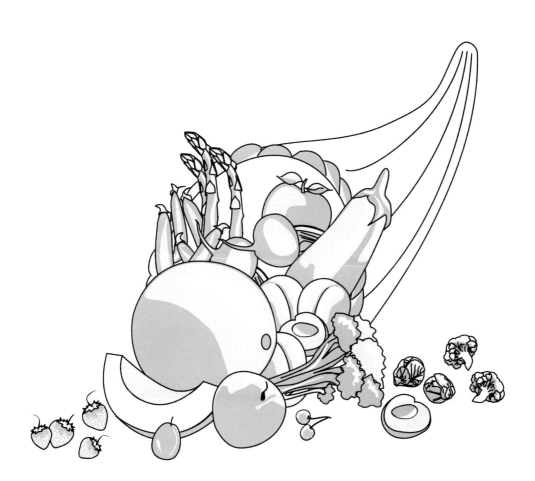

Fresh Baby Recipes

ur recipes are organized according to your baby's age and stage of development. Each chapter includes fruits, vegetables, and proteins. Meats are not included in this book. We do not recommend pureed meats because they are time consuming to prepare and do not appeal to many babies. However, recipes for alternative sources of proteins are included, such as nuts and legumes. In addition, there are no recipes for grains or milk products, as these can be easily purchased at your local grocery or health food store.

Each recipe includes four main topics:

Shopping—This section gives you the information to help select ripe, fresh produce and information on proper storage to preserve freshness.

Nutrition—An easy-to-read 1-, 2-, or 3-star chart shows the nutritional content of each food. Our rating system is based on the USDA Recommended Daily Value of the nutrient and the standard adult serving size.
- 1 star indicates 1-30% of the daily value nutrient in a serving.
- 2 stars indicate 31-60% of the daily value of that nutrient in a serving.
- 3 stars indicate 61% or more of the daily value of that nutrient in a serving.

Cooking—Basic cooking instructions are provided. Variations are also featured for adventurous introductions to more of the flavors your baby will experience in life. Each recipe lists an approximate preparation time—from raw produce to freezer. Most recipes take fewer than 20 minutes to make. If you are using frozen produce, preparation generally requires 5-10 minutes less.

Serving—The Fresh Baby food cube system makes serving meals simple and fast. There is also plenty of room for creativity to make your baby's mealtime a gourmet experience. We recommend tasty food medley combinations that we know go well together. We also encourage you to experiment by combining new foods with one or more of the Fresh Baby recipes to create your own custom medleys for your baby.

Tips to help you on your way

Shopping and Selecting Produce
1: All quantities in the recipes are designed to make at least two Fresh Baby freezer trays.
2: All recipes can be easily cut in half or doubled.
3: All fruit varies in size. If you make too much baby food, you can:
    a: Store the extra in the refrigerator; it will last for 3-4 days.
    b: Store the extra in the refrigerator and freeze it in the trays the next day or when the trays have been emptied.
    c: Use it for the rest of the family—they all taste great and are good for you!
4: Frozen produce: Many grocery stores carry mixtures of fruits and vegetables—these are terrific to use. But before you buy these, make sure you have introduced each ingredient one at a time to ensure there are no allergic reactions to them.

Cook
1: All foods should be at room temperature before cooking. If they are not, cooking time may be longer by 3-5 minutes.
2: Use microwave-safe containers only. The best choices are ceramic and lead-free glass containers or plastic that is specifically labeled "Microwave Safe" or "For Microwave Use."
3: Follow instructions for wrapping or covering food to trap steam.
4: Cooking times: Microwaves vary in power and therefore cooking times might not be exact. Each recipe has a test for doneness. If food is not quite done, try cooking 3-5 minutes longer and let stand another 5 minutes.
5: Standing time: It is very important to observe standing times. Let food remain in the microwave. Microwaves sometimes cook unevenly; standing times allow the cooking process to continue and

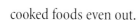

cooked foods even out.

6: Stovetop method: You can prepare all the recipes in this book using a stove, saucepan, and steamer basket. Do not boil food. Follow the same preparation instructions and steam with ½ cup of water in the pan. Reserve remaining liquid in the pan to thin foods—if they need it.

7: When doubling a recipe, cooking time may take longer. Each recipe has a test for doneness. If food is not quite done, try cooking 3-5 minutes longer and let stand another 5 minutes.

Puree

1: At least once during the puree process, stop the appliance and scrape down the sides of the bowl with a spatula.

2: Add water to develop a smooth texture.

   a: Nearly all fruits contain enough juice from cooking and will not need any additional water.

   b: Most vegetables will need additional water. The best way is to add water through the pour hole of a blender or food processor while it is pureeing. If your appliance does not have a pour hole, STOP the appliance, remove the lid, add water, secure the lid, and continue to puree.

   c: Add a little bit of water at time. All vegetables vary in the amount of juice they contain. Start by adding half the recommended water and then a little at a time after that. Sometimes you may need to add a little more than the recommended amount.

   d: When adding water, it is better to be a little thicker in consistency than thinner.

Freeze

1: When possible, let trays cool to room temperature before placing in the freezer.

2: Remove trays from the freezer, pop out the food cubes, and immediately store back in the freezer in storage containers or plastic freezer bags.

3: For easy removal of the food cubes, run warm water on the back of the trays for 5 seconds with the covers still on.

Variations

1: Use herbs, spices, and other flavors in moderation. Remember a little goes a long way in flavoring your baby's foods.

2: Always add any variation ingredient before cooking to allow the flavor to blend with the food that you are cooking.

3: Measurement amounts are for dried herbs and spices. When using fresh herbs, increase the amount: $1/8$ teaspoon of dried is equivalent to one teaspoon of fresh.

The following conversions are approximate. Whichever system you choose, the important thing to remember is to use it throughout the recipe to ensure the proper balance of ingredients. For example, if you start with metric, continue with metric measurements and you'll end up with equivalent proportions of the imperial measurement listed below.

Dry Measures

Imperial	Metric
½ oz.	15g
1 oz	30g
4 oz (¼ lb)	125g
8 oz (½ lb)	250g
12 oz (¾ lb)	375g
16 oz (1lb)	500g
24 oz (1 ½ lb)	750g
32 oz (2lb)	1kg

Liquid Measures

Imperial	Metric	Cup
2 fl oz	60 ml	¼ cup
3 fl oz	90 ml	⅓ cup
4 fl oz	125 ml	½ cup
5 fl oz	150 ml	⅔ cup
6 fl oz	180 ml	¾ cup
8 fl oz	250 ml	1 cup
16 fl oz	500 ml	2 cups
24 fl oz	750 ml	3 cups
32 fl oz	1000 ml (1 litre)	4 cups

Useful Conversions

⅛ teaspoon	0.625 ml
¼ teaspoon	1.25 ml
½ teaspoon	2.5 ml
1 teaspoon	5 ml
1 Australian tablespoon	20 ml (4 teaspoons)
1 UK/US tablespoon	15 ml (3 teaspoons)

First Foods (4-6 months)

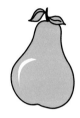

Acorn Squash
Apples
Bananas
Butternut Squash
Green Peas
Pears
Sweet Potatoes

Acorn Squash

Shop

Selection: Look for squash that is heavy for its size, with a dull appearance and hard rind. They should be acorn-shape with deep furrows, green to yellow-gold rind, and yellow flesh.
Storage and ripening: Countertop
Quantity: Fresh—1 large or 2 medium acorn squash. Frozen—2 to 3 10-ounce packages, thawed.

Cook

Step 1 : **Prep** Wash, cut in half, and remove seeds with a spoon. Cut into quarters.
Step 2 : **Cook** Place squash and 2 tablespoons of water in microwave-safe dish. Add ingredients from the Variations list, if desired. Cover with plastic wrap. Cook 10-12 minutes. Let stand 5 minutes. The squash is done when it can be pierced easily with a fork.
Step 3 : **Puree** Scoop out squash meat with a spoon and put into a blender or food processor. Discard skins. Add ½ cup of water. Puree. Add additional ¼ to ½ cup of water, as needed, to develop a smooth texture.
Step 4 : **Pour** Spoon into Fresh Baby trays. Makes 2 trays (24 one-ounce servings).
Step 5 : **Freeze** 8-10 hours or overnight. Remove from trays, place in storage containers or freezer bags, and return immediately to freezer.

Serve

Variations	Age to introduce	Date introduced
⅛ tsp. ground nutmeg	8-10 months	
⅛ tsp. ground cinnamon	8-10 months	
⅛ tsp. ground ginger	8-10 months	
½ tsp. lemon zest	10-12 months	

Select frozen food cubes for the meal, defrost and warm, check the temperature and feed.

Combine with: *	Age to introduce	Liked It?
Apples	4-6 months	
Peaches	6-8 months	
Cauliflower	8-10 months	
Spinach	8-10 months	
1 tsp. ground pecans	8-10 months	
Corn	10-12 months	

* Before making medleys, make sure you introduced each food one at a time.

Nutrition

Protein	—
Potassium	★★
Calcium	★
Iron	★
Vitamin A	★
Vitamin C	★★
Riboflavin	★
Thiamine	★
Niacin	★

Notes: _yucky_

30
Prep Time

Apples

Selection: Select apples that are bruise-free and firm to the touch, with good color (color depends on the variety), flavorful taste, and pleasant smell.

Storage and ripening: Refrigerate. Continues to ripen after harvest. Keep the surface of apples dry. Do not rinse until just before ready to use.

Quantity: 6 medium Golden Delicious apples (sweet) or 3 Golden Delicious and 3 Granny Smith apples (a little tart)

Cook

Step 1: Prep Wash, peel, core, and cut into one-inch slices.

Step 2: Cook Place apples in microwave-safe dish. Add ingredients from the Variations list, if desired. Cover with plastic wrap. Cook 5 minutes and let stand 5 minutes. Cook an additional 5 minutes. The apples are done when they can be pierced easily with a fork.

Step 3: Puree Place apples and cooking juices in a blender or food processor. Puree to a smooth texture.

Step 4: Pour Spoon into Fresh Baby trays. Makes 2 trays (24 one-ounce servings).

Step 5: Freeze 8-10 hours or overnight. Remove from trays, place in storage containers or freezer bags, and return immediately to freezer.

Serve

Variations	Age to introduce	Date introduced
1/8 tsp. ground cinnamon	8-10 months	
1/8 tsp. vanilla extract	8-10 months	
1/8 tsp. ground cloves	8-10 months	
1/8 tsp. ground nutmeg	8-10 months	
1/2 tsp. lemon zest	10-12 months	

Select frozen food cubes for the meal, defrost and warm, check the temperature and feed.

Combine with: *	Age to introduce	Liked It?
Sweet potatoes	4-6 months	
Acorn or butternut squash	4-6 months	
1 Tbsp. yogurt	6-8 months	
Tofu	6-8 months	
1 tsp. ground walnuts	8-10 months	
Berries	10-12 months	

* Before making medleys, make sure you introduced each food one at a time.

Nutrition	
Protein	—
Potassium	*
Calcium	—
Iron	*
Vitamin A	*
Vitamin C	*
Riboflavin	—
Thiamine	*
Niacin	—

Notes: _yummy- but try Mac Intosh_

20 Prep Time

Bananas

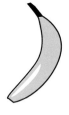

Shop

Selection: Bananas should be of uniform shape and color, regardless of degree of ripeness.
Storage and ripening: Countertop. Continues to ripen after harvest.
Quantity: 1 banana

Cook

Step 1: **Prep** Slice off a piece of banana and peel.

Step 2: **Puree** Mash with fork to a smooth texture. Add ingredients from the Variations list, if desired. Can be thinned with breast milk or formula.

Step 3: **Storage** Can only be used fresh. Save remaining banana by covering the cut end with plastic wrap and store in refrigerator. Before peeling, slice off exposed end that may be a little brown.

Variations	Age to introduce	Date introduced
Sprinkle of ground cinnamon	8-10 months	
1 Tbsp. orange juice	10-12 months	

Serve

Serve at room temperature immediately after preparation.

Combine with: *	Age to introduce	Liked It?
Sweet potatoes	4-6 months	
1 Tbsp. yogurt	6-8 months	
Tofu	6-8 months	
1 tsp. ground pecans	8-10 months	
Cantaloupe	10-12 months	
Berries	10-12 months	

* Before making medleys, make sure you introduced each food one at a time.

Nutrition

Protein	—
Potassium	**
Calcium	—
Iron	*
Vitamin A	—
Vitamin C	*
Riboflavin	*
Thiamine	*
Niacin	*

Notes: _yuck at first then yummy!_

1-2 Prep Time

4-6 Months

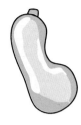

Butternut Squash

Selection: Look for squash that is heavy for its size, with a dull appearance and a hard rind. Butternut squash are large with an elongated, bell shape, tan-colored rind, and yellow-orange flesh.

Storage and ripening: Countertop

Quantity: Fresh—1 medium to large butternut squash. Frozen—2 to 3 10-ounce packages, thawed.

Cook

Step 1 : Prep Wash, cut in half, and remove seeds with a spoon. Cut each half into four pieces.

Step 2 : Cook Place squash and 2 tablespoons of water in a microwave-safe dish. Add ingredients from the Variations list, if desired. Cover with plastic wrap. Cook 10-12 minutes. Let stand 5 minutes. The squash is done when it can be pierced easily with a fork.

Step 3 : Puree Scoop out squash meat with a spoon and put into a blender or food processor. Discard skins. Add fi cup of water. Puree. Add additional ¼ to ½ cup of water, as needed, to develop a smooth texture.

Step 4 : Pour Spoon into Fresh Baby trays. Makes 2 trays (24 one-ounce servings).

Step 5 : Freeze 8-10 hours or overnight. Remove from trays, place in storage containers or freezer bags, and return immediately to freezer.

Serve

Variations	Age to introduce	Date introduced
⅛ tsp. ground nutmeg	8-10 months	
⅛ tsp. ground cinnamon	8-10 months	
⅛ tsp. ground ginger	8-10 months	
½ tsp. lemon zest	10-12 months	

Select frozen food cubes for the meal, defrost and warm, check the temperature and feed.

Combine with: *	Age to introduce	Liked It?
Apples	4-6 months	
Spinach	8-10 months	
1 tsp. ground pecans	8-10 months	
Pineapple	10-12 months	
Corn	10-12 months	

*Before making medleys, make sure you introduced each food one at a time.

30 Prep Time

Notes: 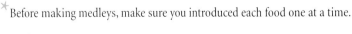 Yummy

Nutrition	
Protein	—
Potassium	*
Calcium	*
Iron	*
Vitamin A	***
Vitamin C	*
Riboflavin	—
Thiamine	*
Niacin	*

Green Peas

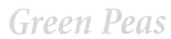

Shop

Selection: All types should have good green color with a soft, velvety touch. Green peas should have well-filled pods with large, round peas.

Storage and ripening: Refrigerate. Pea pods are not edible.

Quantity: Fresh—1 ¾ pounds fresh peas in their pods. Frozen—2 to 3 10-ounce packages, thawed.

Cook

Step 1 : Prep Wash and shell peas. Discard pods.

Step 2 : Cook Place peas and 2 tablespoons of water in a microwave-safe dish. Add ingredients from the Variations list, if desired. Cover with plastic wrap. Cook 6-8 minutes. Let stand 5 minutes. The peas are done when they can be pierced easily with a fork.

Step 3 : Puree Place peas and cooking juices in a blender or food processor and puree. Add ¼ to ½ cup of water, as needed, to develop a smooth texture.

Step 4 : Pour Spoon into Fresh Baby trays. Makes 2 trays (24 one-ounce servings).

Step 5 : Freeze 8-10 hours or overnight. Remove from trays, place in storage containers or freezer bags, and return immediately to freezer.

Variations	Age to introduce	Date introduced
⅛ tsp. dried dill	8-10 months	
¼ sweet onion	8-10 months	
4 button mushrooms	8-10 months	
⅛ tsp. dried tarragon	8-10 months	

Serve

Select frozen food cubes for the meal, defrost and warm, check the temperature and feed.

Nutrition

Protein	*
Potassium	*
Calcium	—
Iron	*
Vitamin A	*
Vitamin C	—
Riboflavin	*
Thiamine	*
Niacin	*

Combine with: *	Age to introduce	Liked It?
Carrots	8-10 months	
White potatoes	8-10 months	
Beets	10-12 months	

* Before making medleys, make sure you introduced each food one at a time.

Notes: _yucky at first then not terribly convinced._

Prep Time 15

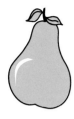

Pears

Selection: Apply gentle thumb pressure near the base of the stem. If it yields slightly, it's ripe.
Storage and ripening: Unripe—countertop in closed paper bag. Ripe—refrigerate. Continues to ripen after harvest.
Quantity: 6 Bartlett or Anjou pears

Cook

Step 1 : **Prep** Wash, cut in half, remove core and skin, and slice into one-inch pieces. Cook immediately or pears will turn brown.

Step 2 : **Cook** Place pears in a microwave-safe dish. Add ingredients from the Variations list, if desired. Cover with plastic wrap. Cook 5 minutes and let stand 5 minutes. The pears are done when they can be pierced easily with a fork.

Step 3 : **Puree** Place pears and cooking juice in a blender or food processor. Puree to a smooth texture.

Step 4 : **Pour** Spoon into Fresh Baby trays. Makes 2 trays (24 one-ounce servings).

Step 5 : **Freeze** 8-10 hours or overnight. Remove from trays, place in storage containers or freezer bags, and place immediately back in freezer.

Serve

Variations	Age to introduce	Date introduced
⅛ tsp. ground ginger	8-10 months	
⅛ tsp. vanilla extract	8-10 months	
½ tsp. lemon or orange zest	10-12 months	

Select frozen food cubes for the meal, defrost and warm, check the temperature and feed.

Combine with: *	Age to introduce	Liked It?
Acorn or butternut squash	4-6 months	
Peas	4-6 months	
Apricots	6-8 months	
Plums	6-8 months	
Peaches	6-8 months	
Berries	10-12 months	

* Before making medleys, make sure you introduced each food one at a time.

15
Prep Time

Notes: _yummy._

Nutrition	
Protein	—
Potassium	★
Calcium	—
Iron	—
Vitamin A	—
Vitamin C	★
Riboflavin	★
Thiamine	—
Niacin	★

Sweet Potatoes/Yams

Selection: Good-quality sweet potatoes should be firm and well-shaped with clean, smooth skins.

Storage and ripening: Countertop

Quantity: 2-3 medium to large sweet potatoes

Cook

Step 1: Prep Wash, peel, and chop into one-inch cubes.

Step 2: Cook Place sweet potatoes/yams and 2 tablespoons of water in a microwave-safe dish. Add ingredients from the Variations list, if desired. Cover with plastic wrap. Cook 8-10 minutes. Let stand 5 minutes. The sweet potatoes/yams are done when they can be pierced easily with a fork.

Step 3: Puree Place sweet potatoes/yams and cooking juices into a blender or food processor. Add ½ cup of water. Puree. Add additional ¼ to ½ cup of water, as needed, to develop a smooth texture.

Step 4: Pour Spoon into Fresh Baby trays. Makes 2 trays (24 one-ounce servings).

Step 5: Freeze 8-10 hours or overnight. Remove from trays, place in storage containers or freezer bags, and return immediately to freezer.

Variations	Age to introduce	Date introduced
⅛ tsp. ground cinnamon	8-10 months	
⅛ tsp. ground cloves	8-10 months	
⅛ tsp. ground ginger	8-10 months	
⅛ tsp. ground nutmeg	8-10 months	

Serve

Select frozen food cubes for the meal, defrost and warm, check the temperature and feed.

Combine with: *	Age to introduce	Liked It?
Apples	4-6 months	
Bananas	4-6 months	
Tofu	6-8 months	
Cauliflower	8-10 months	
1 tsp. ground pecans	8-10 months	

* Before making medleys, make sure you introduced each food one at a time.

Nutrition	
Protein	—
Potassium	★★
Calcium	★
Iron	★
Vitamin A	★★★
Vitamin C	★★
Riboflavin	★
Thiamine	★
Niacin	★

Notes: *Yumny*

30
Prep Time

4-6 Months

6-8 Months

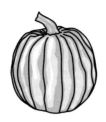

Apricots
Avocados
Green Beans
Nectarines
Peaches
Plums
Pumpkin
Tofu
Yellow Squash
Zucchini

Apricots

Shop

Selection: Look for well-colored, plump apricots with fairly firm texture.
Storage and ripening: Unripe—countertop in a closed paper bag. Ripe—refrigerate. Continues to ripen after harvest.
Quantity: Fresh—12-14 apricots.

Cook

Step 1 **Prep** Wash, cut half, remove pits, and peel.
Step 2 **Cook** Place apricots in a microwave-safe dish. Add ingredients from the Variations list, if desired. Cover with plastic wrap. Cook 3 minutes and let stand 5 minutes. The apricots are done when they can be pierced easily with a fork.
Step 3 **Puree** Place apricots and cooking juices in a blender or food processor. Puree to a smooth texture.
Step 4 **Pour** Spoon into Fresh Baby trays. Makes 2 trays (24 one-ounce servings).
Step 5 **Freeze** 8-10 hours or overnight. Remove from trays, place in storage containers or freezer bags, and return immediately to freezer.

Variations	Age to introduce	Date introduced
⅛ tsp. ground cinnamon	8-10 months	
⅛ tsp. ground nutmeg	8-10 months	

Serve

Select frozen food cubes for the meal, defrost and warm, check the temprerature and feed.

Combine with: *	Age to introduce	Liked It?
1 Tbsp. yogurt	6-8 months	
1 tsp. ground almonds	8-10 months	

* Before making medleys, make sure you introduced each food one at a time.

Nutrition

Protein	—
Potassium	★★
Calcium	★
Iron	★
Vitamin A	★★
Vitamin C	★
Riboflavin	★
Thiamine	★
Niacin	★

Notes: _____

_____

Prep Time 15

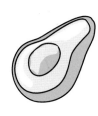

Avocados

Selection: All varieties have green skins; except for Hass avocados, which have a purple-black skin color. Ripe avocados should yield to gentle pressure.

Storage and ripening: Unripe—countertop. Ripe—refrigerate until ready to use. Continues to ripen after harvest.

Quantity: 1 avocado

Cook

Step 1 : **Prep** Slice in half, remove pit, and peel off skin.

Step 2 : **Puree** Mash with a fork to a smooth texture. Add ingredients from the Variations list, if desired.

Step 3 : **Storage** Can only be used fresh. You can save half the avocado by leaving the pit in and keeping the peel on for one day. Cover with plastic wrap and store in the refrigerator.

Variations	Age to introduce	Date introduced
Few drops of lime or lemon juice	10-12 months	

Serve

Serve at room temperature immediately after preparation.

Combine with: *	Age to introduce	Liked It?
Acorn or butternut squash	4-6 months	
1 Tbsp. yogurt	6-8 months	
Tofu	6-8 months	

*Before making medleys, make sure you introduced each food one at a time.

2-3 Prep Time

Notes: _____

_____

Nutrition	
Protein	★
Potassium	★★
Calcium	—
Iron	★
Vitamin A	★
Vitamin C	★
Riboflavin	★
Thiamine	★
Niacin	★

6-8 Months

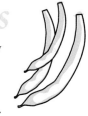

Selection: Good-quality beans should have long, straight pods and be bright green. They should also be free of decay or blemishes and snap easily when bent.

Storage and ripening: Refrigerate. Store unwashed in plastic bags.

Quantity: Fresh—1½ pounds green beans. Frozen—2 to 3 10-ounce packages, thawed.

Cook

Step 1 **Prep** Wash and remove both ends.

Step 2 **Cook** Place green beans and 2 tablespoons of water in a microwave-safe dish. Add ingredients from the Variations list, if desired. Cover with plastic wrap. Cook 8-10 minutes. Let stand 5 minutes. The beans are done when they can be pierced easily with a fork.

Step 3 **Puree** Place green beans and cooking juices in a blender or food processor and puree. Add ¼ to ½ cup of water, as needed, to develop a smooth texture.

Step 4 **Pour** Spoon into Fresh Baby trays. Makes 2 trays (24 one-ounce servings).

Step 5 **Freeze** 8-10 hours or overnight. Remove from trays, place in storage containers or freezer bags, and

6-8 Months

Variations	Age to introduce	Date introduced
4 button mushrooms	8-10 months	
⅛ tsp. dried basil	8-10 months	
½ tsp. lemon zest	10-12 months	

Select frozen food cubes for the meal, defrost and warm, check the temperature and feed.

Combine with: *	Age to introduce	Liked It?
Carrots	8-10 months	
Cauliflower	8-10 months	
White potatoes	8-10 months	
1 tsp. ground almonds	8-10 months	
¼ tsp. ground sesame seeds	8-10 months	
½ ounce soft/semi-hard cheese (one-inch cube), melted	8-10 or 10-12 months	

* Before making medleys, make sure you introduced each food one at a time.

Protein	—
Potassium	*
Calcium	*
Iron	*
Vitamin A	*
Vitamin C	*
Riboflavin	*
Thiamine	*
Niacin	*

Notes: 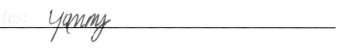 yummy

Prep Time

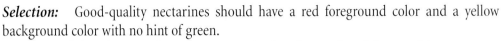

Nectarines

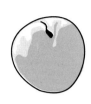

Selection: Good-quality nectarines should have a red foreground color and a yellow background color with no hint of green.

Storage and ripening: Unripe—countertop in closed paper bag. Ripe—refrigerate. Continues to ripen after harvest.

Quantity: 8 nectarines

Cook

Step 1 : Prep Wash, cut in half, and remove pits. Peel and slice into one-inch pieces.

Step 2 : Cook Place nectarines in a microwave-safe dish. Add ingredients from the Variations list, if desired. Cover with plastic wrap. Cook 3 minutes and let stand 5 minutes. The nectarines are done when they can be pierced easily with a fork.

Step 3 : Puree Place nectarines and cooking juices in a blender or food processor. Puree to a smooth texture.

Step 4 : Pour Spoon into Fresh Baby trays. Makes 2 trays (24 one-ounce servings).

Step 5 : Freeze 8-10 hours or overnight. Remove from trays, place in storage containers or freezer bags, and return immediately to freezer.

Serve

Variations	Age to introduce	Date introduced
⅛ tsp. ground cinnamon	8-10 months	
⅛ tsp. ground nutmeg	8-10 months	
⅛ tsp. ground allspice	8-10 months	

Select frozen food cubes for the meal, defrost and warm, check the temperature and feed.

Combine with: *	Age to introduce	Liked It?
Apple	4-6 months	
Pears	4-6 months	
Bananas	4-6 months	
1 tsp. ground walnuts	8-10 months	

* Before making medleys, make sure you introduced each food one at a time.

15 Prep Time

Notes: _____

_____

Nutrition	
Protein	—
Potassium	*
Calcium	—
Iron	*
Vitamin A	*
Vitamin C	*
Riboflavin	*
Thiamine	—
Niacin	*

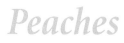

Shop

Selection: Choose bright, fresh-looking peaches. Skin color should be creamy or yellow with varying degrees of red blush or mottling, depending on the variety. Ripe peaches should yield to gentle palm pressure.

Storage and ripening: Unripe—countertop in closed paper bag. Ripe—refrigerate. Continues to ripen after harvest.

Quantity: Fresh—6-7 large peaches. Frozen—2 12 -ounce packages, thawed and peeled.

Cook

Step 1 : **Prep** Wash, cut in half, and remove pits. Peel and cut into one-inch slices.

Step 2 : **Cook** Place peaches in a microwave-safe dish. Add ingredients from the Variations list, if desired. Cover with plastic wrap. Cook 3-5 minutes and let stand 5 minutes. The peaches are done when they can be pierced easily with a fork.

Step 3 : **Puree** Place peaches and cooking juices in a blender or food processor. Puree to a smooth texture.

Step 4 : **Pour** Spoon into Fresh Baby trays. Makes 2 trays (24 one-ounce servings).

Step 5 : **Freeze** 8-10 hours or overnight. Remove from trays, place in storage containers or freezer bags, and return immediately to freezer.

Serve

Variations	Age to introduce	Date introduced
⅛ tsp. ground ginger	8-10 months	
⅛ tsp. ground cinnamon	8-10 months	
⅛ tsp. ground nutmeg	8-10 months	
⅛ tsp. ground allspice	8-10 months	

Select frozen food cubes for the meal, defrost and warm, check the temperature and feed.

Combine with: *	Age to introduce	Liked It?
Apples	4-6 months	
Bananas	4-6 months	
1 Tbsp. yogurt	6-8 months	
1 tsp. ground almonds	8-10 months	
Berries	10-12 months	

* Before making medleys, make sure you introduced each food one at a time.

Notes:
_____
_____

Nutrition

Protein	—
Potassium	∗
Calcium	—
Iron	—
Vitamin A	∗
Vitamin C	∗
Riboflavin	∗
Thiamine	—
Niacin	∗

Prep Time 15

6-8 Months

Plums

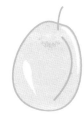

Selection: Plums may be various shades of red, blue, green, and yellow. To test plums for ripeness, apply gentle pressure to the fruit with the thumb and determine if the flesh is beginning to soften.

Storage and ripening: Unripe—countertop. Ripe—refrigerate. Continues to ripen after harvest.

Quantity: 8-10 plums

Cook

Step 1 : Prep Wash, cut in half, and remove pits.

Step 2 : Cook Place plums in a microwave-safe dish. Add ingredients from the Variations list, if desired. Cover with plastic wrap. Cook 5 minutes and let cool. The plums are done when they can be pierced easily with a fork and the skins have pulled away from the meat. Remove and discard the skins.

Step 3 : Puree Place plums and cooking juices in a blender or food processor. Puree to a smooth texture.

Step 4 : Pour Spoon into Fresh Baby trays. Makes 2 trays (24 one-ounce servings).

Step 5 : Freeze 8-10 hours or overnight. Remove from trays, place in storage containers or freezer bags, and return immediately to freezer.

Serve

Variations	Age to introduce	Date introduced
⅛ tsp. ground cinnamon	8-10 months	
½ tsp. orange zest	10-12 months	

Select frozen food cubes for the meal, defrost and warm, check the temperature and feed.

Combine with: *	Age to introduce	Liked It?
Pears	4-6 months	
Peaches	6-8 months	
1 Tbsp. yogurt	6-8 months	

* Before making medleys, make sure you introduced each food one at a time.

20
Prep Time

Notes: *to remove skins quarter slices only skins*

Nutrition	
Protein	—
Potassium	*
Calcium	—
Iron	—
Vitamin A	*
Vitamin C	*
Riboflavin	*
Thiamine	*
Niacin	*

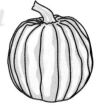

Shop

Selection: Choose clean, well-shaped pumpkins with no cracks in the rind.
Storage and ripening: Countertop
Quantity: 1 small to medium pumpkin

Cook

Step 1 Prep Wash, cut in half, remove seeds with a spoon and discard. Cut each half into four pieces.

Step 2 Cook Place pumpkin and 2 tablespoons of water in microwave-safe dish. Add ingredients from the Variations list, if desired. Cover with plastic wrap. Cook 13-15 minutes. Let stand 5 minutes. The pumpkin is done with it can be pierced easily with a fork.

Step 3 Puree Scoop out pumpkin meat with a spoon and put into a blender or food processor. Discard skins. Add ½ cup of water. Puree. Add an additional ¼ to ½ cup of water, as needed, to develop a smooth texture.

Step 4 Pour Spoon into Fresh Baby trays. Makes 2 trays (24 one-ounce servings).

Step 5 Freeze 8-10 hours or overnight. Remove from trays, place in storage containers or freezer bags, and return immediately to freezer.

Serve

Variations	Age to introduce	Date introduced
⅛ tsp. ground ginger	8-10 months	
⅛ tsp. ground cinnamon	8-10 months	
⅛ tsp. ground nutmeg	8-10 months	

Select frozen food cubes for the meal, defrost and warm, check the temperature and feed.

Combine with: *	Age to introduce	Liked It?
Apples	4-6 months	
Peas	4-6 months	
1 tsp. ground pecans	8-10 months	
Potato	8-10 months	
Cauliflower	8-10 months	

* Before making medleys, make sure you introduced each food one at a time.

Nutrition

Protein	—
Potassium	*
Calcium	*
Iron	*
Vitamin A	***
Vitamin C	*
Riboflavin	*
Thiamine	*
Niacin	*

Notes:
_____
_____

Prep Time

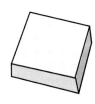

Tofu

Selection: There are two broad categories of tofu—Firm and Soft (or Silken). Silken tofu is best for babies and is eaten raw. Tofu is available in most grocery stores in the produce section.

Storage and ripening: Tofu is like a dairy product in that it must be refrigerated and has a short shelf life. It is normally sold in plastic tubs, immersed in water

Quantity: One small container or tub of soft (silken) tofu

Cook

Step 1 : **Prep** Remove a 2-inch piece of tofu from liquid. Rinse and pat dry with a paper towel.

Step 2 : **Cook** Mash with fork until smooth. Makes a one-ounce serving or about 1 tablespoon.

Step 3 : **Storage** Save remaining tofu and liquid in a covered container. Can be stored in the

Serve

Serve at room temperature immediately after preparation.

Combine with: *	Age to introduce	Liked It?
Acorn or butternut squash	4-6 months	
Avocado	6-8 months	
Spinach	8-10 months	
Berries	10-12 months	

* Before making medleys, make sure you introduced each food one at a time.

Nutrition	
Protein	*
Potassium	*
Calcium	*
Iron	*
Vitamin A	—
Vitamin C	—
Riboflavin	*
Thiamine	*
Niacin	*

30 Prep Time

Notes: _____

_____

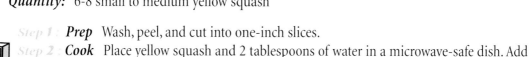

Yellow Squash/Crookneck Squash

Selection: Soft-shell squash should be firm with shiny, tender rinds. Smaller sizes are more tender and flavorful.

Storage and ripening: Refrigerate.

Quantity: 6-8 small to medium yellow squash

Step 1: Prep Wash, peel, and cut into one-inch slices.

Step 2: Cook Place yellow squash and 2 tablespoons of water in a microwave-safe dish. Add ingredients from the Variations list, if desired. Cover with plastic wrap. Cook 8-10 minutes. Let stand 5 minutes. The squash are done when they can be pierced easily with a fork.

Step 3: Puree Place yellow squash and cooking juices in a blender or food processor and puree to a smooth texture. In most cases, no additional water is necessary.

Step 4: Pour Spoon into Fresh Baby trays. Makes 2 trays (24 one-ounce servings).

Step 5: Freeze 8-10 hours or overnight. Remove from trays, place in storage containers or freezer bags, and return immediately to freezer.

Variations	Age to introduce	Date introduced
⅛ tsp. dried dill	8-10 months	
¼ sweet onion	8-10 months	
⅛ tsp. dried chervil	8-10 months	
⅛ tsp. dried marjoram	8-10 months	
⅛ tsp. dried basil	8-10 months	

Select frozen food cubes for the meal, defrost and warm, check the temperature and feed.

Combine with:*	Age to introduce	Liked It?
Peas	4-6 months	
Zucchini	6-8 months	
Green beans	6-8 months	
Cauliflower	8-10 months	

* Before making medleys, make sure you introduced each food one at a time.

Nutrition

Protein	—
Potassium	*
Calcium	*
Iron	*
Vitamin A	*
Vitamin C	*
Riboflavin	*
Thiamine	*
Niacin	*

Notes:
_____
_____

20 Prep Time

6-8 Months

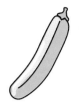

Zucchini

Selection: Soft-shell squash should be firm with shiny, tender rinds. Zucchini is cylindrical in shape, with a shiny, dark green rind. Smaller sizes are more tender and flavorful.

Storage and ripening: Refrigerate.

Quantity: 6-8 small to medium zucchini

Cook

Step 1 : **Prep** Wash, peel, and cut into one-inch slices.

Step 2 : **Cook** Place zucchini and 2 tablespoons of water in a microwave-safe dish. Add ingredients from the Variations list, if desired. Cover with plastic wrap. Cook 8-10 minutes. Let stand 5 minutes. The zucchini is done when it can be pierced easily with a fork.

Step 3 : **Puree** Place zucchini and cooking juices in a blender or food processor and puree to a smooth texture. In most cases, no additional water is necessary.

Step 4 : **Pour** Spoon into Fresh Baby trays. Makes 2 trays (24 one-ounce servings).

Step 5 : **Freeze** 8-10 hours or overnight. Remove from trays, place in storage containers or freezer bags, and return immediately to freezer.

Serve

Variations	Age to introduce	Date introduced
1/8 tsp. dried oregano	8-10 months	
1/8 tsp. dried dill	8-10 months	
1/8 tsp. dried basil	8-10 months	
1/8 tsp. dried marjoram	8-10 months	
1/4 sweet onion	8-10 months	

Select frozen food cubes for the meal, defrost and warm, check the temprerature and feed.

Combine with: *	Age to introduce	Liked It?
Yellow squash	6-8 months	
Carrots	8-10 months	
Cauliflower	8-10 months	
1 tsp. ground walnuts	8-10 months	
Eggplant	10-12 months	

* Before making medleys, make sure you introduced each food one at a time.

Notes: _____

_____

Nutrition	
Protein	—
Potassium	*
Calcium	*
Iron	*
Vitamin A	*
Vitamin C	*
Riboflavin	*
Thiamine	*
Niacin	*

6-8 Months

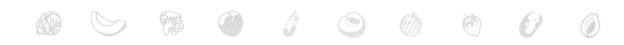

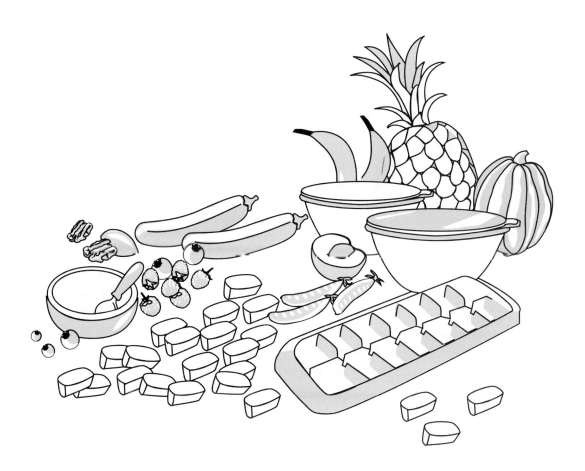

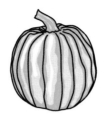

Almonds
Asparagus
Black Beans
Broccoli
Brussels Sprouts
Carrots
Cauliflower
Garbanzo Beans
Mangos
Papayas
Pecans
Pinto Beans
Sesame Seeds
Snow Peas
Spinach
Sugar Snap Peas
Walnuts
White Beans
White Potatoes

Almonds

Shop

Selection: Almonds are available as in-shell, whole shelled, sliced, slivered, diced, and chopped. In-shell nuts should be clean and free of severely damaged or cracked shells.
Storage and ripening: Refrigerate.
Quantity: 4 ounces or ½ cup of shelled almonds

Cook

Step 1 : **Prep**   Crack shells and remove nut meat. Discard shells.
Step 2 : **Puree**   Process in blender until finely ground.
Step 3 : **Pour**   Spoon into storage container. Makes about 36 single-teaspoon servings.
Step 4 : **Freeze**   Freeze. Lasts up to 12 months.

Serve

Add a teaspoon of frozen almonds to baby food.

Combine with *	Age to introduce	Liked It?
Apricots	6-8 months	
Nectarines	6-8 months	
Peaches	6-8 months	
Green beans	6-8 months	
1 Tbsp. yogurt	6-8 months	

*Before making medleys, make sure you introduced each food one at a time.

Nutrition

Protein	**
Potassium	**
Calcium	*
Iron	*
Vitamin A	—
Vitamin C	—
Riboflavin	*
Thiamine	*
Niacin	**

Notes: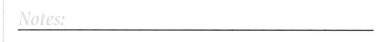

Prep Time 3

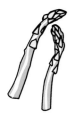

Asparagus

Selection: Asparagus should be fresh and firm with compact tips. Spears should be straight and round, and snap easily when bent. Spears with larger diameters are just as tender as slender spears.

Storage and ripening: Refrigerate. To prolong shelf life, stand asparagus, butt end down, in one inch of water.

Quantity: Fresh—1½ pounds asparagus. Frozen—2 to 3 10-ounce packages, thawed.

Cook

Step 1 : **Prep** Wash, snap off or cut off tough ends, peel stalks, and chop into 2-inch pieces.

Step 2 : **Cook** Place asparagus and 2 tablespoons of water in a microwave-safe dish. Add ingredients from the Variations list, if desired. Cover with plastic wrap. Cook 6-7 minutes and let stand 5 minutes. The asparagus is done when it can be pierced easily with a fork.

Step 3 : **Puree** Place asparagus and cooking juices in a blender or food processor and puree. Add ¼ to ½ cup of water, as needed, to develop a smooth texture.

Step 4 : **Pour** Spoon into Fresh Baby trays. Makes 2 trays (24 one-ounce servings).

Step 5 : **Freeze** 8-10 hours or overnight. Remove from trays, place in storage containers or freezer bags, and return immediately to freezer.

Serve

Variations	Age to introduce	Date introduced
⅛ tsp. dried dill	8-10 months	
⅛ dried chervil	8-10 months	
½ tsp. lemon zest	10-12 months	

Select frozen food cubes for the meal, defrost and warm, check the temperature and feed.

Combine with: *	Age to introduce	Liked It?
Carrots	8-10 months	
Cauliflower	8-10 months	
White potatoes	8-10 months	
½ ounce soft/semi-hard cheese (one-inch cube), melted	8-10 / 10-12 months	

* Before making medleys, make sure you introduced each food one at a time.

Notes:
_____
_____

20 Prep Time

Nutrition

Protein	—
Potassium	*
Calcium	*
Iron	*
Vitamin A	*
Vitamin C	*
Riboflavin	*
Thiamine	*
Niacin	*

Black Beans

Selection: Purchase canned beans that have only a small amount of added salt. Both organic and low-sodium varieties are available. Canned beans are already cooked.

Storage and ripening: Use canned beans within a year of their purchase, sooner if possible, to yield the tastiest product possible.

Quantity: 2 14-ounce cans low-sodium black beans

Cook

Step 1 : ***Prep*** Drain and rinse beans for a least one full minute.

Step 2 : ***Puree*** Place beans and ½ cup of water in a blender or food processor. Add ingredients from the Variations list, if desired. Puree. Add an additional ¼ to ½ cup of water, as needed, to develop a smooth texture.

Step 4 : ***Pour*** Spoon into Fresh Baby trays. Makes 2 trays (24 one-ounce servings).

Step 5 : ***Freeze*** 8-10 hours or overnight. Remove from trays, place in storage containers or freezer bags, and return immediately to freezer.

Serve

Variations	Age to introduce	Date introduced
⅛ tsp. ground cumin	8-10 months	
½ clove of garlic	8-10 months	
⅛ tsp. ground ginger	8-10 months	

Select frozen food cubes for the meal, defrost and warm, check the temperature and feed.

Combine with: *	Age to introduce	Liked It?
Sweet potatoes	4-6 months	
Acorn or butternut squash	4-6 months	
Corn	10-12 months	
½ ounce soft/semi-hard cheese (one-inch cube), melted	8-10 / 10-12 months	

* Before making medleys, make sure you introduced each food one at a time.

Nutrition

Protein	**
Potassium	**
Calcium	*
Iron	*
Vitamin A	—
Vitamin C	—
Riboflavin	*
Thiamine	*
Niacin	*

Notes: _____

_____

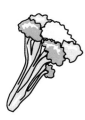

Broccoli

Selection: Good-quality broccoli should have fresh-looking, light green stalks of consistent thickness. Bud clusters should be compact and dark green with a purple tinge.

Storage and ripening: Refrigerate in crisper.

Quantity: Fresh—1 ¾ pounds broccoli. Frozen—2 to 3 10-ounce packages chopped broccoli, thawed.

Cook

Step 1 : Prep Wash, cut off bottoms, and chop into 1-inch pieces.

Step 2 : Cook Place broccoli and 2 tablespoons of water in microwave-safe dish. Add ingredients from the Variations list, if desired. Cover with plastic wrap. Cook 7-10 minutes. Let stand 5 minutes. The broccoli is done when it can be easily pierced with a fork.

Step 3 : Puree Place broccoli and cooking juices in a blender or food processor and puree. Add ¼ to ½ cup of water, as needed, to develop a smooth texture.

Step 4 : Pour Spoon into Fresh Baby trays. Makes 2 trays (24 one-ounce servings).

Step 5 : Freeze 8-10 hours or overnight. Remove from trays, place in storage containers or freezer bags, and return immediately to freezer.

Serve

Variations	Age to introduce	Date introduced
½ clove of garlic	8-10 months	
⅛ tsp. dried dill	8-10 months	
½ tsp. lemon zest	10-12 months	

Select frozen food cubes for the meal, defrost and warm, check the temperature and feed.

Combine with: *	Age to introduce	Liked It?
Carrots	8-10 months	
Cauliflower	8-10 months	
White potatoes	8-10 months	
½ ounce soft/semi-hard cheese (one-inch cube), melted	8-10 / 10-12 months	

* Before making medleys, make sure you introduced each food one at a time.

20 Prep Time

Notes: _____

_____

Nutrition	
Protein	—
Potassium	⋆
Calcium	⋆
Iron	⋆⋆
Vitamin A	⋆⋆
Vitamin C	⋆
Riboflavin	⋆
Thiamine	⋆
Niacin	⋆

Brussels Sprouts

 Shop

Selection: Choose brussels sprouts that are fresh in appearance with good green color. Texture should be firm, leaves compact, and butt ends clean.

Storage and ripening: Refrigerate.

Quantity: Fresh—2 to 3 10-ounce tubs of brussels sprouts. Frozen— 2 to 3 10-ounce packages, thawed.

Cook

Step 1 : Prep Wash, cut off end, and remove outer leaves. Cut in half.

Step 2 : Cook Place brussels sprouts and 2 tablespoons of water in a microwave-safe dish. Add ingredients from the Variations list, if desired. Cover with plastic wrap. Cook 7-9 minutes. Let stand 5 minutes. The brussels sprouts are done when they can be pierced easily with a fork.

Step 3 : Puree Place brussels sprouts and cooking juices in a blender or food processor and puree. Add ¼ to ½ cup of water, as needed, to develop a smooth texture.

Step 4 : Pour Spoon into Fresh Baby trays. Makes 2 trays (24 one-ounce servings).

Step 5 : Freeze 8-10 hours or overnight. Remove from trays, place in storage containers or freezer bags, and return immediately to freezer.

 Serve

Variations	Age to introduce	Date introduced
⅛ tsp. dried dill	8-10 months	
½ tsp. orange or lemon zest	10-12 months	

Select frozen food cubes for the meal, defrost and warm, check the temperature and feed.

Combine with: *	Age to introduce	Liked It?
Sweet potatoes	4-6 months	
Pumpkin	6-8 months	
Carrots	8-10 months	
Corn	10-12 months	

* Before making medleys, make sure you introduced each food one at a time.

Nutrition

Protein	★
Potassium	★★
Calcium	★
Iron	★
Vitamin A	★
Vitamin C	★★★
Riboflavin	★
Thiamine	★
Niacin	★

Notes:

_____

_____

20 Prep Time

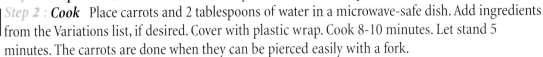

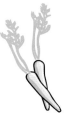

Carrots

Selection: Good-quality carrots should be well-shaped with firm, smooth exteriors. Color should be vibrant orange to orange-red. For best quality, tops should be closely trimmed since they tend to decay rapidly.

Storage and ripening: Refrigerate. Remove green tops and store unwashed in a plastic bag.

Quantity: Fresh—1½ pounds or 10-12 carrots. Frozen—2 to 3 10-ounce packages, thawed.

Cook

Step 1 : Prep Wash, cut off both ends, and peel. Cut into 2-inch pieces.

Step 2 : Cook Place carrots and 2 tablespoons of water in a microwave-safe dish. Add ingredients from the Variations list, if desired. Cover with plastic wrap. Cook 8-10 minutes. Let stand 5 minutes. The carrots are done when they can be pierced easily with a fork.

Step 3 : Puree Place carrots and cooking juices in a blender or food processor and puree. Add ½ to ¾ cup of water, as needed, to develop a smooth texture.

Step 4 : Pour Spoon into Fresh Baby trays. Makes 2 trays (24 one-ounce servings).

Step 5 : Freeze 8-10 hours or overnight. Remove from trays, place in storage containers or freezer bags, and return immediately to freezer.

Serve

Variations	Age to introduce	Date introduced
⅛ tsp. ground ginger	8-10 months	
⅛ tsp. ground cumin	8-10 months	
⅛ tsp. dried dill	8-10 months	
½ tsp. lemon zest	10-12 months	

Select frozen food cubes for the meal, defrost and warm, check the temperature and feed.

Combine with: *	Age to introduce	Liked It?
Peas	4-6 months	
Apples	4-6 months	
Green beans	6-8 months	
White potatoes	8-10 months	
Cauliflower	8-10 months	
Raspberries	10-12 months	

* Before making medleys, make sure you introduced each food one at a time.

Notes:

_____

_____

Nutrition

Protein	—
Potassium	*
Calcium	*
Iron	*
Vitamin A	***
Vitamin C	*
Riboflavin	*
Thiamine	*
Niacin	*

8-10 Months

Shop

Selection: Cauliflower should have creamy white, compact florets with bright green, fresh, and firmly attached leaves. Some small leaves extending through florets do not affect quality.

Storage and ripening: Refrigerate in crisper.

Quantity: Fresh—1 head cauliflower. Frozen—2 to 3 10-ounce packages, thawed.

Cook

Step 1 : Prep Wash, remove all leaves, core and chop florets into 2-inch pieces.

Step 2 : Cook Place cauliflower and 2 tablespoons of water in a microwave-safe dish. Add ingredients from the Variations list, if desired. Cover with plastic wrap. Cook 8-10 minutes. Let stand 5 minutes. The cauliflower is done when it can be pierced easily with a fork.

Step 3 : Puree Place cauliflower and cooking juices in a blender or food processor and puree. Add ½ to ¾ cup of water, as needed, to develop a smooth texture.

Step 4 : Pour Spoon into Fresh Baby trays. Makes 2 trays (24 one-ounce servings).

Step 5 : Freeze 8-10 hours or overnight. Remove from trays, place in storage containers or freezer bags, and return immediately to freezer.

Serve

Variations	Age to introduce	Date introduced
⅛ tsp. dried dill	8-10 months	
¼ sweet onion	8-10 months	
½ tsp. lemon zest	10-12 months	

Select frozen food cubes for the meal, defrost and warm, check the temperature and feed.

Combine with: *	Age to introduce	Liked It?
Acorn or butternut squash	4-6 months	
Peas	4-6 months	
Broccoli	8-10 months	
Carrots	8-10 months	
¼ tsp. ground sesame seeds	8-10 months	
½ ounce soft/semi-hard cheese (one-inch cube), melted	8-10 / 10-12 months	

* Before making medleys, make sure you introduced each food one at a time.

Nutrition	
Protein	—
Potassium	*
Calcium	*
Iron	*
Vitamin A	—
Vitamin C	***
Riboflavin	*
Thiamine	*
Niacin	*

Notes:
_____
_____

Garbanzo Beans/Chick Peas

Shop

Selection: Purchase canned beans that have only a small amount of added salt. Both organic and low-sodium varieties are available. Canned beans are already cooked.
Storage and ripening: Use canned beans within a year of their purchase, sooner if possible, to yield the tastiest product possible.
Quantity: 2 14-ounce cans of low-sodium garbanzo beans.

Cook

Step 1: **Prep** Drain and rinse for a least one full minute.
Step 2: **Puree** Place beans and ½ cup of water in a blender or food processor. Add ingredients from the Variations list, if desired. Puree. Add an additional ¼ to ½ cup of water, as needed, to develop a smooth texture.
Step 4: **Pour** Spoon into Fresh Baby trays. Makes 2 trays (24 one-ounce servings).
Step 5: **Freeze** 8-10 hours or overnight. Remove from trays, place in storage containers or freezer bags, and return immediately to freezer.

Serve

Variations	Age to introduce	Date introduced
1 Tbsp. ground sesame seeds	8-10 months	
½ clove of garlic	8-10 months	
1 Tbsp. lemon juice	10-12 months	

Select frozen food cubes for the meal, defrost and warm, check the temprerature and feed.

Combine with: *	Age to introduce	Liked It?
Peas	4-6 months	
Broccoli	8-10 months	
Asparagus	8-10 months	
Beets	10-12 months	

*Before making medleys, make sure you introduced each food one at a time.

Notes: _____

_____

Prep Time 5

Nutrition

Protein	*
Potassium	*
Calcium	*
Iron	*
Vitamin A	—
Vitamin C	—
Riboflavin	*
Thiamine	*
Niacin	*

8-10 Months

88 | FRESH BABY

Selection: Select full, somewhat firm fruit with taut skin and a strong fragrant aroma.
Storage and ripening: Unripe—countertop. Ripe—refrigerate. Continues to ripen after harvest.
Quantity: Fresh—4 mangos. Frozen—2 12-ounce packages, thawed.

Cook

Step 1 : Prep Wash, cut meat away from the pit, which runs vertically down the middle of the fruit. Peel and cut into one-inch pieces.

Step 2 : Cook Place mangos in a microwave-safe dish. Add ingredients from the Variations list, if desired. Cover with plastic wrap. Cook 3 minutes and let stand 5 minutes. The mangos are done when they can be pierced easily with a fork.

Step 3 : Puree Place mangos and cooking juices in a blender or food processor. Puree to a smooth texture.

Step 4 : Pour Spoon into Fresh Baby trays. Makes 2 trays (24 one-ounce servings).

Step 5 : Freeze 8-10 hours or overnight. Remove from trays, place in storage containers or freezer bags, and return immediately to freezer.

Serve

Variations	Age to introduce	Date introduced
1 tsp. lime or lemon juice	10-12 months	

Select frozen food cubes for the meal, defrost and warm, check the temperature and feed.

Combine with: *	Age to introduce	
Bananas	4-6 months	
Papayas	8-10 months	
Pineapple	10-12 months	
Cantaloupe	10-12 months	

* Before making medleys, make sure you introduced each food one at a time.

Nutrition

Protein	—
Potassium	*
Calcium	—
Iron	—
Vitamin A	**
Vitamin C	**
Riboflavin	*
Thiamine	*
Niacin	*

Notes: _____

_____

Papayas

Selection: Good-quality papayas should be firm with unblemished skins, regardless of degree of ripeness. A papaya is ripe and ready to eat when it yields to gentle palm pressure and the peel is approximately fl yellow to yellow-orange in color.

Storage and ripening: Countertop. Continues to ripen after harvest.

Quantity: Fresh— 4 small papayas or one large papaya. Frozen—2 12-ounce packages, thawed.

Cook

Step 1 : **Prep** Wash, cut in half, remove seeds with spoon and discard. Peel and cut into one-inch slices.

Step 2 : **Cook** Place papaya in a microwave-safe dish. Add ingredients from the Variations list, if desired. Cover with plastic wrap. Cook 3-5 minutes and let stand 5 minutes. The papaya is done when it can be pierced easily with a fork.

Step 3 : **Puree** Place papaya and cooking juices in a blender or food processor. Puree to a smooth texture.

Step 4 : **Pour** Spoon into Fresh Baby trays. Makes 2 trays (24 one-ounce servings).

Step 5 : **Freeze** 8-10 hours or overnight. Remove from trays, place in storage containers or freezer bags, and return immediately to freezer.

Serve

Variations	Age to introduce	Date introduced
1 tsp. lime juice	10-12 months	

Select frozen food cubes for the meal, defrost and warm, check the temprerature and feed.

Combine with: *	Age to introduce	Liked It?
Pears	4-6 months	
Mangos	8-10 months	
Berries	10-12 months	
Pineapple	10-12 months	

* Before making medleys, make sure you introduced each food one at a time.

Notes: _____

_____

Nutrition

Protein	—
Potassium	*
Calcium	*
Iron	*
Vitamin A	*
Vitamin C	***
Riboflavin	*
Thiamine	*
Niacin	*

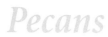
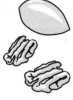

Shop

Selection: Pecans are available in-shell or shelled as whole or half kernels or chopped/diced kernels of various sizes. In-shell nuts should be clean and free of severely damaged or cracked shells.

Storage and ripening: Refrigerate.

Quantity: 4 ounces or ½ cup of shelled pecans.

Cook

Step 1 : **Prep** Crack shells and remove nut meat. Discard shells.
Step 2 : **Puree** Process in blender until finely ground.
Step 3 : **Pour** Spoon into storage container. Makes about 36 single-teaspoon servings.
Step 4 : **Freeze** Freeze. Lasts up to 12 months.

Serve

Add a teaspoon of frozen pecans to baby food.

Combine with: *	Age to introduce	Liked It?
Sweet potatoes	4-6 months	
Acorn or butternut squash	4-6 months	
Pears	4-6 months	
Pumpkin	6-8 months	
1 Tbsp. yogurt	6-8 months	

* Before making medleys, make sure you introduced each food one at a time.

Nutrition

Protein	**
Potassium	**
Calcium	*
Iron	*
Vitamin A	—
Vitamin C	—
Riboflavin	*
Thiamine	*
Niacin	*

Notes:
_____
_____

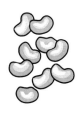

Pinto Beans

Selection: Purchase canned beans that have only a small amount of added salt. Both organic and low-sodium varieties are available. Canned beans are already cooked.

Storage and ripening: Use canned beans within a year of their purchase, sooner if possible, to yield the tastiest product possible.

Quantity: 2 14-ounce cans of low-sodium pinto beans.

Cook

Step 1 : **Prep** Drain and rinse beans for a least one full minute.

Step 2 : **Puree** Place beans and ½ cup of water in a blender or food processor. Add ingredients from the Variations list, if desired. Puree. Add an additional ¼ to ½ cup of water, as needed, to develop a smooth texture.

Step 3 : **Pour** Spoon into Fresh Baby trays. Makes 2 trays (24 one-ounce servings).

Step 4 : **Freeze** 8-10 hours or overnight. Remove from trays, place in storage containers or freezer bags, and return immediately to freezer.

Serve

Variations	Age to introduce	Date introduced
½ sweet onion	8-10 months	
⅛ tsp. ground cumin	8-10 months	
⅛ tsp. curry powder	8-10 months	

Select frozen food cubes for the meal, defrost and warm, check the tempreature and feed.

Combine with: *	Age to introduce	Liked It?
Peas	4-6 months	
Green beans	6-8 months	
Spinach	8-10 months	
Asparagus	8-10 months	
½ ounce soft/semi-hard cheese (one-inch cube), melted	8-10 / 10-12 months	

* Before making medleys, make sure you introduced each food one at a time.

5 Prep Time

Notes: _____

_____

Nutrition	
Protein	⋆
Potassium	⋆
Calcium	⋆
Iron	⋆
Vitamin A	—
Vitamin C	—
Riboflavin	⋆
Thiamine	⋆
Niacin	⋆

8-10 Months

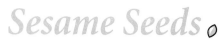

Sesame Seeds

Selection: Sesame seeds are available packaged in the spice section and in bulk quantity in Middle Eastern and health food markets. Tahini, a paste made of ground sesame seeds, can be used in place of ground sesame seeds.

Storage and ripening: Unrefrigerated seeds should be kept in an airtight container in a cool, dry place for up to three months, refrigerated up to six months, or frozen up to one year. Tahini can be refrigerated for up to six months.

Quantity: 1 ounce or about 3 Tablespoons

Cook

Step 1 : ***Puree*** Process in blender until finely ground.

Step 2 : ***Pour*** Spoon into storage container. Makes about 36 ¼-teaspoon servings.

Step 3 : ***Freeze*** Freeze. Lasts up to 12 months.

Serve

Add ¼ teaspoon of frozen sesame seeds to baby food.

Combine with: *	Age to introduce	Liked It?
Snow peas	6-8 months	
Sugar snap peas	6-8 months	
Broccoli	8-10 months	
Cauliflower	8-10 months	

* Before making medleys, make sure you introduced each food one at a time.

Protein	**
Potassium	**
Calcium	**
Iron	**
Vitamin A	—
Vitamin C	—
Riboflavin	*
Thiamine	*
Niacin	**

Notes:
_____
_____

Snow Peas

Selection: All types of peas should have a good green color with a soft, velvety touch. Snow peas should have firm pods.

Storage and ripening: Refrigerate.

Quantity: Fresh—1 ¾ pounds snow peas. Frozen—2 to 3 10-ounce packages, thawed.

Cook

Step 1 : **Prep** Wash and remove both ends.

Step 2 : **Cook** Place snow peas and 2 tablespoons of water in a microwave-safe dish. Add ingredients from the Variations list, if desired. Cover with plastic wrap. Cook 7-9 minutes. Let stand 5 minutes. The peas are done when they can be pierced easily with a fork.

Step 3 : **Puree** Place snow peas and cooking juices in a blender or food processor and puree. Add ¼ to ½ cup of water, as needed, to develop a smooth texture.

Step 4 : **Pour** Spoon into Fresh Baby trays. Makes 2 trays (24 one-ounce servings).

Step 5 : **Freeze** 8-10 hours or overnight. Remove from trays, place in storage containers or freezer bags, and return immediately to freezer.

Serve

Variations	Age to introduce	Date introduced
⅛ tsp. dried dill	8-10 months	
⅛ tsp. dried tarragon	8-10 months	

Select frozen food cubes for the meal, defrost and warm, check the temperature and feed.

Combine with: *	Age to introduce	Liked It?
Carrots	8-10 months	
White potatoes	8-10 months	
¼ tsp. ground sesame seeds	8-10 months	
Beets	10-12 months	

*Before making medleys, make sure you introduced each food one at a time.

Notes:
_____
_____

20 Prep Time

Nutrition	
Protein	—
Potassium	*
Calcium	—
Iron	*
Vitamin A	*
Vitamin C	—
Riboflavin	*
Thiamine	*
Niacin	*

8-10 Months

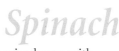

Spinach

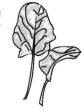

Selection: Good-quality spinach should have clean, fresh, and fairly crisp leaves with good green coloring.

Storage and ripening: Refrigerate in crisper.

Quantity: Fresh—2 pounds spinach. Frozen—2 to 3 10-ounce packages, thawed and squeezed to remove water.

Cook

Step 1 : **Prep** Wash and remove tough stems.

Step 2 : **Cook** Place spinach and 2 tablespoons of water in a microwave-safe dish. Add ingredients from the Variations list, if desired. Cover with plastic wrap. Cook 6-7 minutes. Let stand 5 minutes. The spinach is done when the leaves are wilted.

Step 3 : **Puree** Place spinach and cooking juices in a blender or food processor and puree. Add ¼ to ½ cup of water, as needed, to develop a smooth texture.

Step 4 : **Pour** Spoon into Fresh Baby trays. Makes 2 trays (24 one-ounce servings).

Step 5 : **Freeze** 8-10 hours or overnight. Remove from trays, place in storage containers or freezer bags, and return immediately to freezer.

Serve

Variations	Age to introduce	Date introduced
¼ cup no-salt chicken broth	6-8 months	
¼ sweet onion	8-10 months	
¼ clove of garlic	8-10 months	
¼ cup coconut milk	10-12 months	

Select frozen food cubes for the meal, defrost and warm, check the temperature and feed.

Combine with: *	Age to introduce	Liked It?
Sweet potatoes	4-6 months	
Butternut or acorn squash	4-6 months	
White potatoes	8-10 months	
½ ounce soft/semi-hard cheese (one-inch cube), melted	8-10 / 10-12 months	

*Before making medleys, make sure you introduced each food one at a time.

Nutrition

Protein	—
Potassium	**
Calcium	*
Iron	*
Vitamin A	**
Vitamin C	*
Riboflavin	*
Thiamine	*
Niacin	*

Notes: _____

_____

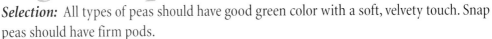

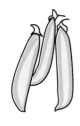

Sugar Snap Peas

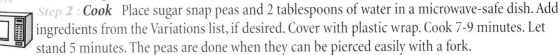

Selection: All types of peas should have good green color with a soft, velvety touch. Snap peas should have firm pods.

Storage and ripening: Refrigerate.

Quantity: Fresh—1 ¾ pounds sugar snap peas. Frozen— 2 to 3 10-ounce packages, thawed.

Cook

Step 1 : Prep Wash and remove both ends.

Step 2 : Cook Place sugar snap peas and 2 tablespoons of water in a microwave-safe dish. Add ingredients from the Variations list, if desired. Cover with plastic wrap. Cook 7-9 minutes. Let stand 5 minutes. The peas are done when they can be pierced easily with a fork.

Step 3 : Puree Place sugar snap peas and cooking juices in a blender or food processor and puree. Add ¼ to ½ cup of water, as needed, to develop a smooth texture.

Step 4 : Pour Spoon into Fresh Baby trays. Makes 2 trays (24 one-ounce servings).

Step 5 : Freeze 8-10 hours or overnight. Remove from trays, place in storage containers or freezer bags, and return immediately to freezer.

Serve

Variations	Age to introduce	Date introduced
⅛ tsp. dried dill	8-10 months	
⅛ tsp. dried tarragon	8-10 months	

Select frozen food cubes for the meal, defrost and warm, check the temperature and feed.

Combine with: *	Age to introduce	Liked It?
Carrots	8-10 months	
White potatoes	8-10 months	
¼ tsp. ground sesame seeds	8-10 months	
Beets	10-12 months	

* Before making medleys, make sure you introduced each food one at a time.

20 Prep Time

Notes: _____

_____

Nutrition	
Protein	—
Potassium	*
Calcium	—
Iron	*
Vitamin A	*
Vitamin C	—
Riboflavin	*
Thiamine	*
Niacin	*

8-10 Months

Walnuts

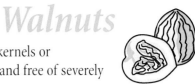

Shop

Selection: Walnuts are available in-shell or shelled as whole or half kernels or chopped/diced kernels of various sizes. In-shell nuts should be clean and free of severely damaged or cracked shells.

Storage and ripening: Refrigerate.

Quantity: 4 ounces or ¼ cup of shelled walnuts

Cook

Step 1 : **Prep**   Crack shells and remove nut meat. Discard shells.

Step 2 : **Puree**   Process in blender until finely ground.

Step 3 : **Pour**   Spoon into storage container. Makes about 36 single-teaspoon servings.

Step 4 : **Freeze**   Freeze. Lasts up to 12 months.

Serve

Add a teaspoon of frozen walnuts to baby food.

Combine with: *	Age to introduce	Liked It?
Apples	4-6 months	
Pears	4-6 months	
Zucchini	6-8 months	
1 Tbsp. yogurt	6-8 months	

* Before making medleys, make sure you introduced each food one at a time.

Nutrition

Protein	**
Potassium	**
Calcium	*
Iron	*
Vitamin A	—
Vitamin C	—
Riboflavin	*
Thiamine	*
Niacin	*

Notes:
_____

_____

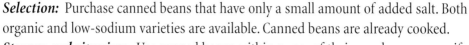

White Beans

Shop

Selection: Purchase canned beans that have only a small amount of added salt. Both organic and low-sodium varieties are available. Canned beans are already cooked.

Storage and ripening: Use canned beans within a year of their purchase, sooner if possible, to yield the tastiest product possible.

Quantity: 2 14-ounce cans of low-sodium white beans

Cook

Step 1 : **Prep** Drain and rinse beans for a least one full minute.

Step 2 : **Puree** Place beans and ½ cup of water in a blender or food processor. Add ingredients from the Variations list, if desired. Puree. Add additional ¼ to ½ cup of water, as needed, to develop a smooth texture.

Step 3 : **Pour** Spoon into Fresh Baby trays. Makes 2 trays (24 one-ounce servings).

Step 4 : **Freeze** 8-10 hours or overnight. Remove from trays, place in storage containers or freezer bags, and return immediately to freezer.

Serve

Variations	Age to introduce	Date introduced
⅛ tsp. dried tarragon	8-10 months	
⅛ tsp. ground ginger	8-10 months	
½ clove of garlic	8-10 months	

Select frozen food cubes for the meal, defrost and warm, check the temperature and feed.

Combine with: *	Age to introduce	Liked It?
Acorn or butternut squash	4-6 months	
Peas	4-6 months	
Green beans	6-8 months	
Spinach	8-10 months	

*Before making medleys, make sure you introduced each food one at a time.

Notes: _____

_____

Prep Time 5

Nutrition

Protein	★★
Potassium	★★
Calcium	★
Iron	★
Vitamin A	—
Vitamin C	—
Riboflavin	★
Thiamine	★
Niacin	★

8-10 Months

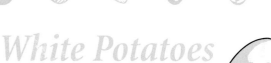

White Potatoes

Selection: All potato varieties should be uniformly sized, fairly clean, firm, and smooth.
Storage and ripening: Countertop.
Quantity: 2 to 3 large Idaho or baking potatoes.

Cook

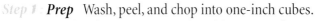

Step 1 : **Prep** Wash, peel, and chop into one-inch cubes.
Step 2 : **Cook** Place potatoes and 2 tablespoons of water in a microwave-safe dish. Add ingredients from the Variations list, if desired. Cover with plastic wrap. Cook 8-10 minutes. Let stand 5 minutes. The potatoes are done when they can be easily pierced with a fork.
Step 3 : **Puree** Place potatoes and cooking juices in a blender or food processor. Add ½ cup of water. Puree. Add an additional ¼ to ½ cup of water, as needed, to develop a smooth texture.
Step 4 : **Pour** Spoon into Fresh Baby trays. Makes 2 trays (24 one-ounce servings).
Step 5 : **Freeze** 8-10 hours or overnight. Remove from trays, place in storage containers or freezer bags, and return immediately to freezer.

Serve

Variations	Age to introduce	Date introduced
½ clove of garlic	8-10 months	
⅛ tsp. dried rosemary	8-10 months	
¼ sweet onion	8-10 months	

Select frozen food cubes for the meal, defrost and warm, check the temperature and feed.

Combine with: *	Age to introduce	Liked It?
Sweet potatoes	4-6 months	
Green beans	6-8 months	
Peas	6-8 months	
Carrots	8-10 months	
½ ounce soft/semi-hard cheese (one-inch cube), melted	8-10 / 10-12 months	

* Before making medleys, make sure you introduced each food one at a time.

Nutrition

Protein	*
Potassium	**
Calcium	*
Iron	*
Vitamin A	—
Vitamin C	**
Riboflavin	*
Thiamine	*
Niacin	*

Notes: _____

_____

Beets
Blueberries
Cantaloupe
Cherries
Corn
Dates
Eggplant
Pineapple
Raspberries
Strawberries

Selection: Choose small to medium beets with firm, smooth skins and purple-red color.
Storage and ripening: Refrigerate.
Quantity: Fresh—8 medium beets. Frozen—2 to 3 10-ounce packages, thawed.

Step 1 **Prep** Wash and cut off top and root end. Peel and cut into one-inch slices. Wear gloves or the beets will discolor your hands.

Step 2 **Cook** Place beets and 2 tablespoons of water in a microwave-safe dish. Add ingredients from the Variations list, if desired. Cover with plastic wrap. Cook 10-12 minutes. Let stand 5 minutes. The beets are done when they are pierced easily with a fork.

Step 3 **Puree** Place beets and liquid in a blender or food processor and puree. Add ¼ to ½ cup of water, as needed, to develop a smooth texture.

Step 4 **Pour** Spoon into Fresh Baby trays. Makes 2 trays (24 one-ounce servings).

Step 5 **Freeze** 8-10 hours or overnight. Remove from trays, place in storage containers or freezer bags, and place immediately back in freezer.

Variations	Age to introduce	Date introduced
⅛ tsp. dried dill	8-10 months	
½ tsp. orange zest	10-12 months	

Select frozen food cubes for the meal, defrost and warm, check the temperature and feed.

Combine with: *	Age to introduce	Liked It?
Apples	4-6 months	
Sweet potatoes	4-6 months	
1 Tbsp. yogurt	6-8 months	
Carrots	8-10 months	
White potatoes	8-10 months	

* Before making medleys, make sure you introduced each food one at a time.

Protein	—
Potassium	*
Calcium	*
Iron	*
Vitamin A	—
Vitamin C	*
Riboflavin	*
Thiamine	*
Niacin	*

Notes:
_____
_____

Blueberries

Shop

Selection: Plump, juicy berries with a deep purple to blue-black skin color highlighted by a silvery sheen called "bloom."

Storage and ripening: Refrigerate. Does not ripen after harvest.

Quantity: Fresh—1 ½ pounds blueberries. Frozen—2 12-ounce packages, thawed.

Cook

Step 1: Prep Wash and remove any stems or debris.

Step 2: Cook Place blueberries in a microwave-safe dish. Add ingredients from the Variations list, if desired. Cover with plastic wrap. Cook 3 minutes and let stand 5 minutes. The berries are done when they are juicy and can be mashed easily with a fork.

Step 3: Puree Place blueberries and cooking juices in a blender or food processor. Puree to a smooth texture.

Step 4: Pour Spoon into Fresh Baby trays. Makes 2 trays (24 one-ounce servings).

Step 5: Freeze 8-10 hours or overnight. Remove from trays, place in storage containers or freezer bags, and return immediately to freezer.

Serve

Variations	Age to introduce	Date introduced
⅛ tsp. ground cinnamon	8-10 months	
⅛ tsp. ground nutmeg	8-10 months	
½ tsp. lemon zest	10-12 months	

Select frozen food cubes for the meal, defrost and warm, check the temperature and feed.

Combine with: *	Age to introduce	Liked It?
Pears	4-6 months	
Apples	4-6 months	
Bananas	4-6 months	
1 Tbsp. yogurt	6-8 months	

*Before making medleys, make sure you introduced each food one at a time.

Notes: _____

_____

Nutrition

Protein	—
Potassium	—
Calcium	*
Iron	*
Vitamin A	—
Vitamin C	*
Riboflavin	*
Thiamine	*
Niacin	*

10-12 Months

15 Prep Time

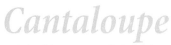

Cantaloupe

Selection: A ripe cantaloupe will have a distinctive aroma and the blossom end should yield to gentle pressure.

Storage and ripening: Uncut—countertop. Cut—refrigerate. Does not ripen further after harvest.

Quantity: 1 medium to large cantaloupe.

Cook

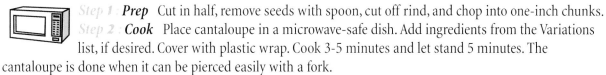

Step 1 **Prep** Cut in half, remove seeds with spoon, cut off rind, and chop into one-inch chunks.

Step 2 **Cook** Place cantaloupe in a microwave-safe dish. Add ingredients from the Variations list, if desired. Cover with plastic wrap. Cook 3-5 minutes and let stand 5 minutes. The cantaloupe is done when it can be pierced easily with a fork.

Step 3 **Puree** Place cantaloupe and cooking juices in a blender or food processor. Puree to a smooth texture.

Step 4 **Pour** Spoon into Fresh Baby trays. Makes 2 trays (24 one-ounce servings).

Step 5 **Freeze** 8-10 hours or overnight. Remove from trays, place in storage containers or freezer bags, and place immediately back in freezer.

Variations	Age to introduce	Date introduced
Few drops of lime or lemon juice	10-12 months	

Serve

Select frozen food cubes for the meal, defrost and warm, check the temperature and feed.

Combine with: *	Age to introduce	Liked It?
Bananas	4-6 months	
Papayas	8-10 months	
Mangos	8-10 months	

* Before making medleys, make sure you introduced each food one at a time.

Nutrition

Protein	—
Potassium	*
Calcium	—
Iron	*
Vitamin A	**
Vitamin C	***
Riboflavin	*
Thiamine	*
Niacin	*

Notes:

_____

_____

15 Prep Time

10-12 Months

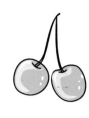

Cherries

Selection: Look for cherries that are plump with firm, smooth, and brightly colored skins. Good-quality cherries should have green stems attached.

Storage and ripening: Refrigerate. Does not ripen further after harvest. Cherries bruise easily; handle with care.

Quantity: Fresh—1½ pounds sweet cherries. Frozen—2 12-ounce packages, thawed.

Cook

Step 1 : **Prep** Wash, cut in half, and remove pit.

Step 2 : **Cook** Place cherries in a microwave-safe dish. Add ingredients from the Variations list, if desired. Cover with plastic wrap. Cook 3 minutes and let stand 5 minutes. The cherries are done when they can be pierced easily with a fork.

Step 3 : **Puree** Place cherries and cooking juices in a blender or food processor. Puree to a smooth texture.

Step 4 : **Pour** Spoon into Fresh Baby trays. Makes 2 trays (24 one-ounce servings).

Step 5 : **Freeze** 8-10 hours or overnight. Remove from trays, place in storage containers or freezer bags, and return immediately to freezer.

10-12 Months

Serve

Variations	Age to introduce	Date introduced
⅛ tsp. ground cinnamon	8-10 months	

Select frozen food cubes for the meal, defrost and warm, check the temperature and feed.

Combine with: *	Age to introduce	Liked It?
Apples	4-6 months	
Pears	4-6 months	
1 tsp. ground walnuts	8-10 months	

*Before making medleys, make sure you introduced each food one at a time.

Notes: _____

_____

20 Prep Time

Nutrition

Protein	—
Potassium	*
Calcium	*
Iron	*
Vitamin A	*
Vitamin C	**
Riboflavin	*
Thiamine	*
Niacin	*

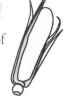

Corn

Selection: Good-quality corn should have fresh green husks with silk ends that are free of decay or worms. Ears should be evenly covered with plump, consistently sized kernels.
Storage and ripening: Refrigerate. Corn is highly perishable; eat as soon as possible.
Quantity: Fresh—8 ears of corn. Frozen— 2 to 3 10-ounce packages, thawed.

Cook

Step 1 : **Prep** Remove husk, wash, and cut kernels off the cob.
Step 2 : **Cook** Place corn and 2 tablespoons of water in a microwave-safe dish. Add ingredients from the Variations list, if desired. Cover with plastic wrap. Cook 6-7 minutes. Let stand 5 minutes.
Step 3 : **Puree** Place corn and cooking juices in a blender or food processor and puree. Add ¼ to ½ cup of water, as needed, to develop a smooth texture.
Step 4 : **Pour** Spoon into Fresh Baby trays. Makes 2 trays (24 one-ounce servings).
Step 5 : **Freeze** 8-10 hours or overnight. Remove from trays, place in storage containers or freezer bags, and place immediately back in freezer.

Serve

Variations	Age to introduce	Date introduced
¼ sweet onion	8-10 months	
⅛ tsp. dried dill	8-10 months	
⅛ tsp. dried marjoram	8-10 months	

Select frozen food cubes for the meal, defrost and warm, check the temperature and feed.

Combine with: *	Age to introduce	Liked It?
Acorn and butternut squash	4-6 months	
Apples	4-6 months	
Peas	4-6 months	
Green beans	6-8 months	

* Before making medleys, make sure you introduced each food one at a time.

Nutrition

Protein	*
Potassium	*
Calcium	—
Iron	*
Vitamin A	*
Vitamin C	*
Riboflavin	*
Thiamine	*
Niacin	*

Notes:
_____
_____

Prep Time

Dates

Selection: Pitted dried dates are recommended for this recipe.
Storage and ripening: Refrigerate.
Quantity: 16-18 dried pitted dates.

Cook

Step 1 : **Prep** If dates are not pitted, cut in half and remove pits.

Step 2 : **Cook** Place dates in a microwave-safe dish with ¾ cup of water. Add ingredients from the Variations list, if desired. Cover with plastic wrap. Cook 7-9 minutes and let stand 5 minutes. The dates are done when they are plump and can be easily mashed with a fork.

Step 3 : **Puree** Place dates and cooking juices in a blender or food processor. Puree to a smooth texture.

Step 4 : **Pour** Spoon into Fresh Baby trays. Makes 2 trays (24 one-ounce servings).

Step 5 : **Freeze** 8-10 hours or overnight. Remove from trays, place in storage containers or freezer bags, and return immediately to freezer.

Serve

Variations	Age to introduce	Date introduced
⅛ tsp. ground ginger	8-10 months	
⅛ tsp. ground cinnamon	8-10 months	

Select frozen food cubes for the meal, defrost and warm, check the temperature and feed.

Combine with: *	Age to introduce	Liked It?
Bananas	4-6 months	
1 Tbsp. yogurt	6-8 months	
1 tsp. ground walnuts	8-10 months	

* Before making medleys, make sure you introduced each food one at a time.

Nutrition	
Protein	—
Potassium	✦✦
Calcium	✦
Iron	✦
Vitamin A	—
Vitamin C	—
Riboflavin	✦
Thiamine	✦
Niacin	✦✦

20 Prep Time

Notes: _____
_____

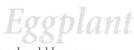

Eggplant

Selection: Look for firm eggplants that are light for their size. Skin should be even-colored and free of blemishes.

Storage and ripening: Refrigerate.

Quantity: Fresh—2-3 medium to large eggplants.

Cook

Step 1 : Prep Wash, peel, and cut into one-inch cubes.

Step 2 : Cook Place eggplant and 2 tablespoons of water in a microwave-safe dish. Add ingredients from the Variations list, if desired. Cover with plastic wrap. Cook 8-10 minutes. Let stand 5 minutes. The eggplant is done when it can be pierced easily with a fork.

Step 3 : Puree Place eggplant and cooking juices in a blender or food processor and puree to a smooth texture. In most cases, no additional water is necessary.

Step 4 : Pour Spoon into Fresh Baby trays. Makes 2 trays (24 one-ounce servings).

Step 5 : Freeze 8-10 hours or overnight. Remove from trays, place in storage containers or freezer bags, and place immediately back in freezer.

Variations	Age to introduce	Date introduced
⅛ tsp. dried oregano	8-10 months	
⅛ tsp. dried basil	8-10 months	
⅛ tsp. dried marjoram	8-10 months	

Serve

Select frozen food cubes for the meal, defrost and warm, check the temperature and feed.

Combine with: *	Age to introduce	Liked It?
Zucchini	6-8 months	
Yellow squash	6-8 months	
¼ tsp. sesame seeds	8-10 months	

* Before making medleys, make sure you introduced each food one at a time.

Nutrition

Protein	—
Potassium	*
Calcium	—
Iron	*
Vitamin A	—
Vitamin C	*
Riboflavin	*
Thiamine	—
Niacin	*

Notes:
_____
_____

Prep Time

10-12 Months

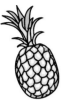

Pineapple

Selection: Pineapples should be heavy for their size, well-shaped, and fresh-looking with dark green crown leaves. Shells should be dry, crisp, and range in color from greenish-brown to golden brown.

Storage and ripening: Refrigerate. Does not ripen further after harvest.

Quantity: Fresh—1 medium pineapple. Frozen—2 12-ounce packages.

Cook

Step 1: **Prep** Wash. Cut off skin, remove core, and cut into one-inch chunks.

Step 2: **Cook** Place pineapple in a microwave-safe dish. Add ingredients from the Variations list, if desired. Cover with plastic wrap. Cook 5 minutes and let stand 5 minutes. The pineapple is done when it can be pierced easily with a fork.

Step 3: **Puree** Place pineapple and cooking juices in a blender or food processor. Puree to a smooth texture.

Step 4: **Pour** Spoon into Fresh Baby trays. Makes 2 trays (24 one-ounce servings).

Step 5: **Freeze** 8-10 hours or overnight. Remove from trays, place in storage containers or freezer bags, and return immediately to freezer.

Serve

Variations	Age to introduce	Date introduced
⅛ tsp. ground cinnamon	8-10 months	

Select frozen food cubes for the meal, defrost and warm, check the temperature and feed.

Combine with: *	Age to introduce	Liked It?
Bananas	4-6 months	
Peas	4-6 months	
Papayas	8-10 months	
Mangos	8-10 months	
Berries	10-12 months	

*Before making medleys, make sure you introduced each food one at a time.

15
Prep Time

Notes: _____

_____

Nutrition

Protein	—
Potassium	*
Calcium	—
Iron	—
Vitamin A	—
Vitamin C	*
Riboflavin	*
Thiamine	—
Niacin	*

10-12 Months

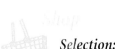

Shop

Selection: Good-quality raspberries should be dry, plump, and firm.
Storage and ripening: Refrigerate. Raspberries are highly perishable and should be used within 1-2 days after purchase.
Quantity: Fresh—1½ pounds raspberries. Frozen—2 12-ounce packages, thawed.

Step 1 Prep Wash and remove any stems or debris.
Step 2 Cook Place raspberries in a microwave-safe dish. Add ingredients from the Variations list, if desired. Cover with plastic wrap. Cook 3 minutes and let stand 5 minutes. The berries are done when they are juicy and can be mashed easily with a fork.
Step 3 Puree Place raspberries and cooking juices in a blender or food processor. Puree to a smooth texture.
Step 4 Pour Spoon into Fresh Baby trays. Makes 2 trays (24 one-ounce servings).
Step 5 Freeze 8-10 hours or overnight. Remove from trays, place in storage containers or freezer bags, and place immediately back in freezer.

Serve

Variations	Age to introduce	Date introduced
½ tsp. lemon or orange zest	10-12 months	

Select frozen food cubes for the meal, defrost and warm, check the temperature and feed.

Combine with: *	Age to introduce	Liked It?
Apples	4-6 months	
Pears	4-6 months	
Bananas	4-6 months	
1 Tbsp. yogurt	6-8 months	

* Before making medleys, make sure you introduced each food one at a time.

Protein	—
Potassium	★
Calcium	★
Iron	★
Vitamin A	—
Vitamin C	★★
Riboflavin	★
Thiamine	★
Niacin	★

Notes:
_____
_____

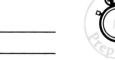

10-12 Months

Strawberries

Selection: Strawberries should be plump and firm with a bright red color and natural shine. Caps should be fresh, green, and intact.

Storage and ripening: Refrigerate. Does not ripen further after harvest. Do not wash berries until just before use.

Quantity: Fresh—1½ pounds strawberries. Frozen—2 12-ounce packages, thawed.

Cook

Step 1 : **Prep** Wash, remove green stem and white core.

Step 2 : **Cook** Place strawberries in a microwave-safe dish. Add ingredients from the Variations list, if desired. Cover with plastic wrap. Cook 3 minutes and let stand 5 minutes. The berries are done when they are juicy and can be pierced easily with a fork.

Step 3 : **Puree** Place strawberries and cooking juices in a blender or food processor. Puree to a smooth texture.

Step 4 : **Pour** Spoon into Fresh Baby trays. Makes 2 trays (24 one-ounce servings).

Step 5 : **Freeze** 8-10 hours or overnight. Remove from trays, place in storage containers or freezer bags, and return immediately to freezer.

Serve

Variations	Age to introduce	Date introduced
¼ cup orange juice	10-12 months	
½ tsp. orange zest	10-12 months	

Select frozen food cubes for the meal, defrost and warm, check the temperature and feed.

Combine with: *	Age to introduce	Liked It?
Bananas	4-6 months	
1 Tbsp. yogurt	4-6 months	
Apples	4-6 months	
Pears	4-6 months	
Peaches	6-8 months	

* Before making medleys, make sure you introduced each food one at a time.

15 Prep Time

Notes:
_____
_____

Nutrition	
Protein	—
Potassium	*
Calcium	*
Iron	*
Vitamin A	—
Vitamin C	***
Riboflavin	*
Thiamine	*
Niacin	*

10-12 Months

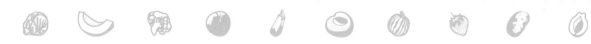

Recipe index (alphabetical)

Topic index (alphabetical)